K-H

Alcohol-Related Misconduct

Blackacre Series on Discipline and Discharge

Alcohol-Related Misconduct

Adolph M. Koven
Susan L. Smith

Coloracre Publications, Inc.
San Francisco, California

KENDALL/HUNT
PUBLISHING COMPANY
Dubuque, Iowa

Library of Congress Catalog Card Number: 84–81022

ISBN 0–8403–3329–3

Printed in the United States of America

B 403329 01

To John Scalone, Larry Corbett, Michael Lehmann, Ed Miller, and Don MacIntyre for their encouragement and sober criticism.

CONTENTS

INTRODUCTION

"JUST CAUSE"—WHAT DOES IT MEAN?

The number and types of employee misconduct are many indeed, but there is only one accepted standard by which the propriety of discipline or discharge for misconduct is measured: the principle of *just cause*. Nearly every labor agreement contains a provision that an employee may be discharged or disciplined only for just cause (or one of its alter egos, such as "proper cause," "good cause," or just plain "cause"). A trend has been developing in the courts, too, to recognize an individual employee's right to protest his dismissal through legal channels even in the absence of a collective bargaining agreement based on his claim that "just cause" was not present.[1]

But commonplace as the term "just cause" may be, it is easily one of the most frustrating concepts to management, especially first-line supervisors.

Why? Because the just-cause standard cannot be defined exactly, as arbitrators have recognized for a long time.[2] It has been referred to as the "introduction of civil rights into the labor agreement"; as what "the reasonable man" would say was an equitable basis for discipline; as simply a "fair shake." The problem with definitions like this is that they are too general to be of much use in deciding whether discipline is warranted in a particular case. When it comes down to cases, a more practical approach is needed.

Such a practical approach has been concretized in a set of seven tests or standards, originally formulated by Arbitrator Carroll Daugherty in the celebrated case of *Enterprise Wire Co.*, 46 LA 362 (1966), and widely applied by arbitrators. In these seven standards, Daugherty

[1]Summers, "Individual Protection against Unjust Dismissal: Time for a Statute," 62 VIRGINIA L. REV., 481, 500 (1976).

[2]"There is no absolute answer to the question what constitutes just or sufficient cause for discharge. . . ." (*Waste King Corp.*, 66–1 ARB ¶8007 (Hon, 1966); "To be sure, no standards exist to aid an arbitrator in finding a conclusive answer to such a question. . . ." (*Riley Stoker Corp.*, 7 LA 767 (1947).

gathered together the basic elements of just cause emphasized by different arbitrators and translated them into a working method for determining when there is just cause for discipline.

1. NOTICE: "Did the Employer give to the employee forewarning or foreknowledge of the possible or probable consequences of the employee's disciplinary conduct?"
2. REASONABLE RULE OR ORDER: "Was the Employer's rule or managerial order reasonably related to (a) the orderly, efficient, and safe operation of the Employer's business, and (b) the performance that the Employer might properly expect of the employee?"
3. INVESTIGATION: "Did the Employer, *before* administering the discipline to an employee, make an effort to discover whether the employee did in fact violate or disobey a rule or order of management?"
4. FAIR INVESTIGATION: "Was the Employer's investigation conducted fairly and objectively?"
5. PROOF: "At the investigation, did the "judge" obtain substantial evidence or proof that the employee was guilty as charged?"
6. EQUAL TREATMENT: "Has the Employer applied its rules, orders and penalties even-handedly and without discrimination to all employees?"
7. PENALTY: "Was the degree of discipline administered by the Employer in a particular case reasonably related to (a) the seriousness of the employee's *proven* offense, and (b) the record of the employee in his service with the Employer?"

JUST CAUSE AND ALCOHOL-RELATED MISCONDUCT

What just cause means and how it has been applied by arbitrators and other labor relations professionals is explored in detail in the volume JUST CAUSE: THE SEVEN TESTS (Koven and Smith, Coloracre Publications, 1985) in which "the basics" of each of the seven tests are analyzed. For example, the chapter on "Notice" covers matters common to all varieties of misconduct, such as whether notice must be given in writing that certain conduct is prohibited; what are the typical pitfalls that an employer is likely to encounter with notice issues; when notice is not necessary. Under Reasonable Rules, the question of who decides what is "reasonable," among other matters, is discussed; Investigation helps the reader find his way through the controversy over whether the rights against self-incrimination and unreasonable search and seizure that employees enjoy in private life carry over into the workplace.

The scope of ALCOHOL-RELATED MISCONDUCT is both broader and narrower than the volume on JUST CAUSE. It is narrower in the sense that it takes the larger principles developed in JUST CAUSE as its foundation and does not itself develop those principles in detail. But it expands those principles as they relate specifically to discipline for alcohol-related misconduct.

The purpose of this book is to familiarize the manager and the supervisor as well as the union representative and the shop steward and others interested in the labor-management field with how arbitrators have applied the seven just-cause standards in cases involving alcohol violations. While every disciplinary action is subject to just-cause criteria, each type of employee misconduct presents its own special problems with reference to the seven Daugherty tests.

In alcohol cases, Notice normally is not a decisive factor, except in a few specific areas—where, for example, the employer intends to require employees suspected of intoxication to take sobriety tests. The second test, the Reasonable Rule test, is also not an issue in cases of intoxication, drinking, or possession of alcohol on company premises, but comes into play with discipline for off-premises drinking and chronic alcoholism.

On the other hand, Investigation and Fair Investigation, Proof, Equal Treatment, and Penalty, either independently or in connection with one another, all may play major roles in just-cause discipline for alcohol-related offenses, and the ways in which these tests typically come up in cases of this type are explored in detail below. Interrelationships among the seven tests are also discussed, and several are highlighted in boxes titled "The Connection."

PROOF AND ALCOHOL-RELATED MISCONDUCT

Throughout ALCOHOL-RELATED MISCONDUCT, references also appear to sections in another volume in the Blackacre Series on Discipline and Discharge: PROOF AND EVIDENCE IN DISCIPLINE AND

DISCHARGE (Koven and Smith, Coloracre Publications, 1985). For example, highlights from the chapter on hearsay include: what is meant when hearsay is admitted "for what it is worth;" when hearsay is not hearsay ("Exceptions to the Hearsay Rule"); and "Hearsay's Main Hurdles." The chapter on circumstantial evidence, among other topics, gives the reader "Nine Keys to the World of Circumstantia," while the chapter on credibility explores such subjects as the guidelines by which credibility can be gained or lost as well as the pros and cons of the "Shulman connection."

HOW TO USE THIS BOOK

ALCOHOL-RELATED MISCONDUCT is mainly intended for managers and supervisors at every level at which drinking problems must be confronted at the workplace, in grievance handling, and in arbitration. Secondarily, it is also directed to lawyers on both sides of the aisle, to shop stewards and other union representatives, and to students of labor relations and the arbitration process.

Basically there are three aspects to this material:

First, as a general treatment of the three main categories of alcohol violations, i.e., intoxication, drinking, and possession of alcoholic beverages, as well as the special disciplinary problems that relate to the chronic alcoholic—for short-hand purposes call it *the overall aspect*.

Next, as a guide to determining what kind of action to take when the company is confronted with an actual rule violation—call it *the how-to aspect*. For analyzing a particular case of alcohol-related misconduct to determine whether the seven just-cause tests have been satisfied, a Final Checklist appears on p. 158. The last section of this checklist deals with the chronic alcoholic.

Finally, as a resource for those who want to know what the authorities in the field have to say—call it *the lawyerly aspect*.

Odds and Ends

• The research on which this volume is based has focused primarily upon arbitration cases decided within the last 10 years, though "lead cases" may be drawn from prior years.

• The SUPPOSEs and EXAMPLEs which appear in the text are based upon actual cases. To the extent that they highlight certain aspects of those cases, and do not reproduce the facts in their entirety, they might be called "reasonable facsimiles" of those cases rather than "absolute facsimiles."

The names have been changed so that in every case the grievant is named "Harry Workman" or "Helen Workman"; the first-line supervisor, "Miles Foreman"; second-line supervisor, "Ed Leader"; the personnel manager or other upper management representative, "Dave Powers"; and other employees, "Mike Armstrong" and "Arnie Hammer."

• The book contains two case lists. The first, Appendix A, "Key Cases—With Topics Covered," is organized according to the four areas of intoxication, drinking, possession, and chronic alcoholism. The second list, Appendix B, "Key Cases in Detail," sets forth the facts of six lead cases on drinking and intoxication and how the arbitrator analyzed and decided each case using principles drawn from the seven just-cause tests.

• Finally, Appendix C is a bibliography listing books and articles to which the reader may refer for additional information on this critical area of labor-management relations.

Chapter 1

NOTICE

"Did the Employer give to the employee forewarning or foreknowledge of the possible consequences of the employee's disciplinary conduct?"

Arbitrator Koven: "[I]t is well recognized that before an employee can be justifiably disciplined for a breach of an employer's rules or regulations, he must have knowledge of the rule or regulation which he is charged with violating."[1]

TWO COMPONENTS: MISCONDUCT AND ITS CONSEQUENCES

"Forewarning" and "foreknowledge" mean "Notice"—i.e., the employer's responsibility to communicate to employees *what it considers to be misconduct* and *what penalties will result* from particular acts of misconduct *before* any penalty actually is imposed. The most important single feature of the "Notice" test in reference to alcohol-related misconduct is that it is not a serious problem *except* in the area of penalty.

First Component: Misconduct

Virtually every company has a rule or contract provision which prohibits the three major categories of alcohol-related misconduct, i.e., intoxication, drinking, and possession of alcoholic beverages in the workplace. And even in the unlikely event that a company had no rule spelling out that employees could be disciplined for alcohol violations, employees are expected to know, even without the existence of a rule, that drinking and working do not mix.

[1]*Bay Area Rapid Transit District,* 80–2 ARB ¶8612 (1980).

Arbitrator Keltner: "[A] Company does not have to establish that it had, or that it had communicated specific rules for certain well-recognized proven offenses such as drunkenness, theft, or insubordination. . . ."[2]

Because notice is a matter of common sense in alcohol cases, the employer does not have to concern himself about many of the typical notice pitfalls into which he may stumble when he tries to discipline employees for less obvious varieties of misconduct; questions like "Was the company's rule specifically worded enough to tell employees what was expected of them?" simply do not apply.

Thus in one case where the union argued that a rule against "drinking on duty" was too vague to be enforced, and if taken literally would prevent employees from drinking even water or soda pop, the arbitrator dismissed that argument as "patently absurd." Everyone in the industrial community knows, he found, that "the word 'drinking' when used in a prohibiting context connotes and is limited to the drinking of intoxicants."[3] And everyone knows additionally that the drinking of intoxicants can lead to discipline.

One exception: off-premises misconduct

SUPPOSE: *Private lives*

Harry Workman, who is employed as a common laborer, is convicted in municipal court of drunken driving and promptly discharged by the company. The union protests that Workman was on his own time when he was arrested, was driving his own car, and was not engaged in any business for the company. But the company claims it has a long-established rule providing for discharge of an employee convicted of driving while intoxicated and that all employees are advised of that rule when they are hired.

This case raised not one but two separate notice questions. *First,* had the rule been clearly communicated to the grievant and other employees? Not certain, the arbitrator decided. The company itself admitted that the rule had never been reduced to writing and posted on the bulletin board, and the grievant denied that any supervisor had ever informed him about the rule orally.

[2]*Philco Corp.*, 45 LA 437 (1965).

[3]*Browning-Ferris Industries of Ohio, Inc.*, 77 LA 289, 292 (Shanker, 1981).

Second, did the rule give clear notice that it would be applied to employees in their private lives? No, the arbitrator said, explaining:

> "Since as a matter of 'common law' applicable to industrial relations, what an employee does on his own time is not subject of regulation by the employer, any qualifying restriction *must be expressly set out in clear and unequivocal language.* In the absence of any such language evidencing a contrary intent, it must be concluded that the language, such as the foregoing, was designed and intended to regulate and apply to employees during working hours."

The conclusion: Since Workman was not on notice that his off-premises conduct could get him fired, his discharge was set aside.[4]

Express notice might not be required if off-premises, off-clock drinking had such a direct effect on the employer's business that an employee should know that discipline would be warranted. Suppose, in the foregoing example, that Workman had been driving a borrowed company truck when he was arrested—he might as well whistle "Dixie" as argue that "no one ever told him" such conduct would result in discipline. (For other types of situations in which drinking off-premises so directly affects the employer's business that notice is not an issue—and other situations where notice is necessary—see Chapter 2, "Reasonable Rules.")

Another special problem area: blood alcohol tests

Notice may also enter the picture if the employer seeks to use the results of a blood alcohol test (otherwise known as a "sobriety test") to prove that an employee is under the influence. In some cases, where the company had not informed employees in advance that anyone suspected of being intoxicated might be required to submit to testing, arbitrators have held that an employee has the right to say, "Thanks, but no thanks," without being penalized for his refusal. (See Chapter III, "Investigation.")[5]

[4]*Lamb Glass Co.,* 32 LA 420, 423 (Dworkin, 1959) (emphasis added). No back pay was awarded because the grievant failed to give required notice that he would be unable to report for work while he was being held in jail following his arrest.

[5]See *Greif Brothers Corp.,* KEY CASES IN DETAIL, where the company had neither informed employees in advance that rejection of a sobriety test might be taken as proof of intoxication nor determined in advance the procedures according to which tests would be conducted. Lack of notice was also a key consideration in *Capital Area Transit Authority,* 69 LA 811, 815 (Ellman, 1977), where the blood-test requirement was communicated by a "secret" memorandum to supervisory personnel only, and not to employees or to the union. "In such circumstances, grievant was under no obligation to comply with the Authority's direction. Whatever may have been the amount of his alcoholic consumption . . . if any, his discharge lacked just cause."

Advance notice might also be required if the company decided to select a particular blood alcohol percentage (0.10 percent—the level of "intoxication" under many state motor vehicle codes—or some other percentage) as automatic proof of intoxication.

FOR EXAMPLE:

Although an employee scored 0.14 percent and 0.15 percent on two successive blood alcohol tests, his discharge for intoxication was set aside. Reason: The employer decided only after the test results were in that the blood alcohol level would be the standard for measuring intoxication. Employees are entitled to be told what criteria the company intends to use *before* it takes action against them, the arbitrator stated. Had the grievant known that a sobriety test would be required and how the results would be interpreted, he might have elected to stay home that day instead of placing his job in jeopardy.[6]

A major problem with setting standards after the fact is that the employer is vulnerable to the charge that he was "out to get" someone and tailor-made a definition of intoxication to fit a particular situation. If a standard is announced in advance, and is applied to all employees consistently, no suspicion of discrimination is likely to arise.[7]

Second Component of Notice: Penalty

The majority of notice problems in alcohol cases relate to the question of penalty, especially for drinking and possession of alcohol. The notice test, as arbitrators have generally understood it, means that the company must let employees know not only what kinds of conduct will lead to discipline, but *what sort of discipline* is likely to result.

Notice of the penalty that the employee risks by engaging in certain misconduct is particularly important if the penalty in question is discharge. Even in cases where employees have engaged in clearly un-

[6]*Northrop Worldwide Aircraft Services, Inc.*, 64 LA 742 (Goodstein, 1975). See also *Lockheed Aircraft Corp.*, 28 LA 829, 831 (Hepburn, 1957): "The Company can probably declare that liquor on an employee's breath, without more, constitutes just cause for suspension or discharge, but *unless this is known to employees* (or should have been known) a discharge for this and nothing more is not just cause. The Company states that a certain percentage of alcohol in the blood constitutes proof of being under the influence of alcohol, and is just cause, but *if this meaning has not been communicated to an employee*, it is not just cause in his case." (Emphasis added.)

[7]As, for example, in *Day & Zimmerman*, KEY CASES IN DETAIL, where the company uniformly used a blood alcohol level of 0.10 percent as proof of intoxication and discharged every employee who met or exceeded that standard.

acceptable conduct and therefore been subject to *some* penalty, arbitrators have put them back to work if they were not forewarned that discharge could be the consequence.

> *Arbitrator Ipavec:* "An occasion for discipline is not necessarily an appropriate occasion for discharge. The Employee should be aware of the significance which the Company attaches to a prohibited act and, in a case of disobedience, that the sanction will be immediate discharge."[8]

Reasonable expectations

Even if company rules explicitly prohibit drinking and possession, as well as intoxication, many employees might not believe the company would view a drink or two as seriously as full-blown intoxication. Especially if the drink happens to be beer (which is often consumed simply as a thirst-quencher and not necessarily for its intoxicating properties), common-sense notions about the relative "harmlessness" of limited drinking may lead an employee to think that if he is caught drinking on the job, he may get a slap on the wrist or perhaps a suspension, but nothing as drastic as discharge.

Many arbitrators, too, believe that drinking and possession are lesser violations than intoxication (see "Penalty," p. 128); or at least accept the fact that employees may see things that way. For that reason, discharge for a first offense of drinking or possession has often been thrown out if employees have not been explicitly warned that drastic consequences *can* result from "minor" violations.

SUPPOSE: *"How was I to know?"*

Cocktail waitress Helen Workman is discharged after she drinks a beer during the course of her shift. The union agrees that Workman's conduct was improper but argues that employees have never been put on notice that one drink could lead to discharge. Written company rules make discharge the penalty for a first offense of drunkenness on duty, and the company contends that employees are informed orally at the time of hire that drinking, too, is a dischargeable offense. Union witnesses dispute that contention.

The arbitrator began with the proposition that drinking is not as inherently wrong as on-the-job drunkenness and then reasoned in two steps: "[I]f the employer is going to prohibit and discharge for drinking on the job, he best have a rule on the subject"; and "if he has such a

[8]*Gray Drug Stores, Inc.*, 53 LA 1329, 70–1 ARB ¶8115 (1969)

rule, he obviously has to properly notify and apprise the employees of such a rule." Because of the conflicting testimony on whether "oral notice" was given, the arbitrator was not persuaded that Workman knew that her conduct could lead to discharge, and she was reinstated without back pay.[9]

Suppose, on the other hand, that either company rules or the contract itself states up front that discharge is reserved for a first offense of intoxication, and specifies some other penalty for drinking or possession. That would amount to indirect notice that discharge will *not* result from those lesser infractions, and employees would be entitled to rely on that notice.

Where, for example, the contract required the company to give an employee at least one warning prior to suspension or discharge, except in the case of dishonesty, being under the influence of narcotics or intoxicating beverages, willful destruction of company property and a few other serious offenses, the arbitrator found that the company was barred from discharging an employee for a first offense of alcohol possession; the contractually required warning was substituted for discharge, and the employee was awarded back pay.[10]

"May, might, must"

There is a world of difference between rules that state in no uncertain terms that discharge is mandatory for alcohol-related offenses and rules that say employees "may be discharged" or "are subject to discharge" for the same misconduct. Variations on "may" and "might"

[9]*Riverview Supper Club*, 82–2 ARB ¶8467 (Jacobowski, 1982). See also *Wagner Electric Corp.*, 57 LA 11, 72–1 ARB ¶8027 (Erbs, 1971) (drinking eliminated as cause for summary discharge in recent revision of company rules; employees no longer on notice they could be fired for drinking); *Altamil Corp.*, 71–1 ARB ¶8198 (Volz, 1971) (no notice that drinking a beer on a break could lead to discharge); *Trans World Airlines*, 38 LA 1221 (Wallen, 1962) (discharge for violating rule against drinking within 12 hours of reporting for duty not mandatory under company rules; *Red Arrow Freight Lines, Inc.*, 78 LA 141 (Baron, 1982) (rule must state that discharge is mandatory if discharge for first offense of possession is to be upheld; *Anvan Industries, Inc.*, 72–2 ARB ¶8516 (Kossoff, 1972) (notice that drinking is subject to summary discharge does not apply to possession).

[10]*National Car Rental System, Inc.*, 75 LA 518 (Zumas, 1980). Similarly, *Baumfolder Corp.*, 78 LA 1060 (Modjeska, 1982), where the grievant's discharge for reporting to work under the influence was reduced to the two-day suspension set forth in company rules. In *Northwest Airlines, Inc.*, 56 LA 837, 71–1 ARB ¶8346 (Wyckoff, 1971), "drunkenness or possession of liquor on job" was listed in company rules among "more serious violations" justifying immediate discharge. Since the rule against drinking alcohol within 24 hours before reporting to work was not included in that "more serious" category, the arbitrator concluded that something short of discharge must have been contemplated for a first offense and reinstated the grievants with two-month suspensions.

and "could be" dilute the effect of notice to the extent that an employee may be left somewhat uncertain as to the consequences of misconduct, even misconduct as serious as intoxication. An arbitrator might then jump into the breach and revoke a discharge on the ground that the company never gave notice of how seriously it viewed the infraction in question.

Nevertheless, more flexible language may benefit the employer as well as the employee.

THE CONNECTION—In re: Penalty

By avoiding notice that certain penalties are mandatory for alcohol-related misconduct, the employer leaves himself elbow room to exercise reasonable discretion, e.g., to consider an employee's length of service, performance record, and other factors that may play a part in fashioning a proper penalty.[11]

[11]*Continental Can Co.*, 68–2 ARB ¶8785, 5726 (Dworkin, 1968): "[T]he rule itself recognizes that an offense 'may' be cause for immediate dismissal, which suggests that immediate dismissal would not automatically follow for every violation of the rule where it is the first offense. The language of the rule contemplates that the determination of the penalty shall result from the exercise of sound discretion on the part of management." In *Altamil Corp.*, 71–1 ARB ¶8198 (Volz, 1971), the arbitrator found that a unilaterally adopted company rule which listed discharge as the penalty for possession of or drinking alcohol on company premises at any time had to be interpreted in the light of the contract's just-cause provision. Discharge could therefore not be applied mechanically without taking into account the relative seriousness of an employee's offense and other mitigating circumstances.

Chapter 2

REASONABLE RULES

"Was the Employer's rule or managerial order reasonably related to (a) the orderly, efficient and safe operation of the Employer's business, and (b) the performance that the Employer might properly expect of the employee?"

INTRODUCTION

Unless exceptional circumstances prevail, everyone knows as a matter of common sense that an employee cannot drink spirits on the job even if there are not any rules that say so right out. Thus, written (and unwritten) rules against intoxication, drinking and possession of alcohol on company premises,[1] or reporting to work under the influence, are routinely endorsed by arbitrators as being "reasonable," and the employer's business needs in reference to the sanctions against on-the-job alcohol use have been spelled out many times. As in the case of "Notice," few cases of discipline for alcohol-related misconduct falter because the company rule involved does not meet the test of reasonableness.

> *Arbitrator Smith:* "The man who deliberately drinks on the job . . . not only steals time which properly belongs to the employer, and contributes to a breakdown in plant morale by his open flouting of the rules; in addition, his condition may reach the point, before he is noticed by supervision, where he seriously endangers other employees or the employer's property."[2]

[1]Rules against intoxication, etc., also routinely cover off-company premises where employees are "on the job," as in the case of truck drivers, servicemen, or salesmen.

[2]*McInerney Spring & Wire Co.*, 21 LA 80, 82 (R. Smith, 1953).

Arbitrator Ellman: "[M]anagement certainly has abundant justification in requiring employees to give full attention to their jobs, unclouded by alcohol or drugs, and soberly to maintain productivity, and assure their own safety and that of fellow employees, as well as to protect company property. The prohibition in Rule 2 that garage employees shall not 'report for work under the influence of alcohol' is clearly reasonable. . . ."[3]

A PREVIEW

Reasonableness problems *do arise* in connection with no-alcohol rules in three general areas:

I. Unreasonable Application of a Reasonable Rule
- Possession and intent
- On premises, but off the clock

II. Drinking Off the Clock, Off Company Premises
- Seven critical conditions

III. The Case of the Chronic Alcoholic
- What is a chronic alcoholic? nine criteria
- Enter the question of just cause: illness v. misconduct

I. UNREASONABLE APPLICATION OF A REASONABLE RULE

While rules against the use of alcohol on company premises are uniformly held to be proper and reasonable, on occasion the *application* of those rules has been called into question.

POSSESSION AND INTENT

The application of rules against having spirits in one's possession or bringing alcoholic beverages onto company premises is particularly susceptible to challenge. Unlike drinking or intoxication, possession may sometimes prove to be "innocent."

[3]*Capital Area Transit Authority,* 69 LA 811, 813 (Ellman, 1977).

SUPPOSE: "I didn't mean to do it."

Harry Workman has an almost empty bottle of vodka in the glove compartment of his car, which is parked on the company lot; the vodka is left over from a recent fishing trip. During the shift, Arnie Hammer mentions that he could sure use a drink, and Workman tells him there is a bottle in his car. Hammer goes and gets the bottle and sets it down on a table a few feet away from Workman. Miles Foreman spots the bottle, establishes that it belongs to Workman, and discharges him.

The outcome: The case turns on the proposition that "mental attitude or intent" is part of an offense, and that the kind of possession which company rules prohibit is "the kind of possession which is likely to lead to drinking on the premises." *First, the car:* Since there was only a small amount of vodka in the bottle (confirming Workman's "fishing trip" explanation), and since there was no evidence that Workman intended drinking on company property, the arbitrator concludes that his "possession" of the vodka in his car was not the kind of possession that amounted to "misconduct" under company rules. No penalty was therefore called for. *Second, the plant:* Nor was Workman technically "in possession" of the bottle, since it was Hammer who brought it into the plant. Had the bottle Hammer retrieved been for their joint use, Workman, too, might have been guilty. But that was not the case. No misconduct on Workman's part, and therefore no penalty.

But Workman was guilty of one offense: making intoxicating liquor available to Hammer. For that reason, no back pay was awarded.[4]

Caveat: Where an employee makes a plausible claim that he brought alcohol to work unknowingly (a flask in a coat pocket left over from an evening's drinking the night before); or that he brought it in to drink after working hours (an unopened bottle of wine stored in a locker or a car for an after-work party), the company may have to prove that he intended to drink it on the premises if any penalty at all (especially a serious one) is to stick.[5]

[4]*Philip Morris, Inc.*, 68–2 ARB ¶8773 (Volz, 1968). The arbitrator elaborated further, "If an employee brings an intoxicant into the plant in his lunch bucket . . . it may be presumed that his intent is to consume the contents on the premises. The situation is otherwise, however, where the intoxicant is found in an automobile . . . [which] is used for transportation, and in the usual case, it is as consistent to presume that liquor and beer found in a vehicle will be used off premises as that they will be consumed thereon."

[5]As in *Packaging Corp. of America*, 56 LA 856 (Anrod, 1971) (grievant had forgotten about bottle she had taken from her car and placed in her purse the night before); *Holcroft Co.*, 55 LA 907 (Keefe, 1970) (whiskey bottle "planted" in grievant's car).

ON PREMISES, BUT OFF THE CLOCK

SUPPOSE:

Young Harry Workman has a little too much to drink one night and as a lark, enters company property without authorization and drives his motorcycle through the plant. The company fires him for violating plant rules against horseplay and appearing on the premises under the influence of alcohol.

The union protests that because Workman was on his own time on the night in question, the company could not properly apply its work rules to him and had no reasonable excuse to penalize him.[6]

The union's argument, of course, doesn't wash—at least not completely. Clocking out doesn't put an end to an individual's status as an employee, and when he is on its premises, the company has a right to expect him to follow the rules—especially rules intended for the protection of people and property.

So the company had every right to throw the book at Workman. His actions not only were extremely dangerous to employees and to the company's product (plate glass) but were "calculated to impair and to undermine the authority of management in its relationship with its employees." Workman escaped discharge solely because of his good work record and the arbitrator's conviction that he had learned his lesson.

But under different circumstances, the "off-clock" factor may have a mitigating effect on the penalty.

SUPPOSE:

Harry Workman and Mike Armstrong meet at a local tavern after work and have a few drinks to celebrate Armstrong's birthday. Armstrong happens to mention his belief that two other employees, Debs and Hammer, are angry with Workman. Workman disagrees and, to prove his point, proposes that they go back to the plant and get Debs and Hammer to have a drink with them.

Workman and Armstrong drive into the plant, park at the dock and locate their friends. The rendezvous is short-lived, however—a supervisor, who happens on the scene, tells Workman and Armstrong to leave and the next day both are fired for being intoxicated on company

[6] *Pittsburgh Plate Glass Co.*, 49 LA 370, 67–2 ARB ¶8559 (Dworkin, 1967).

premises, inducing other employees to drink, and entering the plant without authorization.[7]

In this case the outcome was dictated by the absence of the usual reasons why no-alcohol rules may be enforced by the company, on or off the clock: "The men did not lose time from work. They did not become belligerent, boisterous, nor use loud or vulgar language. They did not endanger the safety or personnel or property. They were celebrating a birthday."

For those reasons, and because it was not clear that the grievants had invited other employees to drink with them *on the premises,* discharge was too harsh—though a suspension was imposed for entering the plant without authorization.

II. DRINKING OFF COMPANY PREMISES

No discipline is warranted *unless* one or more of the following "seven critical conditions" that link an employee's off-premises drinking to his job is present:

1. Drinking *off* premises leads to an employee's showing up *on* premises under the influence.
2. Off-premises drinking results in an unauthorized absence or other work-related misconduct.
3. The drinker has a company vehicle in his custody when he's drinking off the clock.
4. The drinker is a truck driver (or bus driver, etc.) who gets into trouble for mixing drinking and driving.
5. The company has a rule covering alcohol use immediately before work or during breaks.
6. The employer's public image is at stake.
7. An employee has had previous difficulties because of chronic alcoholism and his continued employment depends on his remaining strictly "on the wagon."

[7]*Weatherhead Co.,* 54 LA 158 (Volz, 1969). See also *Conner Manufacturing Co.,* 63 LA 1102 (Mulhall, 1974), in which discharge was held to be too severe for an employee who was allowed to clock out after some lunch hour drinking, and was terminated after he later returned to the plant, allegedly intoxicated, at what he believed had been the request of his supervisor; and *Pennsylvania Greyhound Bus Co.,* 18 LA 400 (1952), where discharge was too severe a penalty for a bus driver who violated a rule prohibiting intoxication on company premises, since the premises in question were a company-owned dormitory, driver was off duty, and he could not be seen by the public.

It is well established that what an employee does when he is off company premises, and not on company time, is his own business and not his employer's. Thus an employee's off-the-clock drinking (like any other aspect of his personal life) cannot normally be considered "misconduct" that would be subject to any form of discipline.

There are exceptions to that general rule, however, as Arbitrator Ferguson pointed out in his frequently cited *Inland Container Corp.*, 28 LA 312, 314 (1957):

> "While it is true that the employer does not become the guardian of the employee's every personal action and does not exercise parental control, it is equally true that *in those areas having to do with the employer's business,* the employer has the right to terminate the relationship *if the employee's wrongful actions injuriously affect the business.*
>
> "The connection between the facts which occur and the extent to which the business is affected must be reasonable and discernible. They must be such as could logically be expected to cause some result measured on its own merits."(Emphasis added.)

The questions then become: What are "those areas having to do with the employer's business"? And, in what ways might an "employee's wrongful actions injuriously affect the business"?

DRINKING OFF PREMISES: SEVEN CRITICAL CONDITIONS

Discipline for off-premises drinking generally breaks down into seven major categories, based on the nature of the connection between the employee's drinking and his job. *Discipline becomes reasonable WHEN:*

Condition No. 1: Drinking OFF premises leads to an employee's showing up ON premises under the influence (the "spill-over" type of case)

The majority of off-premises drinking cases are covered by this condition. What is subject to penalty is not off-premises drinking *per se,* but an employee's inability to work as a result of (say) a few beers at lunch or a stop at the local tavern before his shift—a state of affairs that's very much the employer's business. The issue in this type of case, then, is not Reasonableness but proof and degree of penalty.

Condition No. 2: Off-premises drinking results in an unauthorized absence or other work-related misconduct.

SUPPOSE:

Harry Workman, an airline fleet service clerk, is discharged after he misses a day's work while sleeping off a night's drinking binge in jail and fails to call the company to report his absence. The union pleads that Workman should be excused because his physical condition prevented him from working or making a phone call.

A reasonable excuse? Far from it. Once intoxicated to the point of passing out, Workman may not have been able to report his absence, but the choice of whether to get so drunk that he could not go to work was his choice alone. Especially since Workman's past attendance record was poor, this final demonstration of indifference to his responsibilities amply justified his discharge.[8]

This second condition is obviously similar to the "spill-over" condition, in that it isn't off-clock drinking *per se* that leads to discipline but the fact that, with a kind of domino effect, it prevents an employee from showing up for work or causes him to violate some other rule or policy. Typical types of misconduct to which off-clock drinking may lead:

- Unauthorized or unexcused absence[9]
- Excessive absenteeism[10]
- Destruction of company property[11]

[8]*American Airlines, Inc.*, 46 LA 737 (Sembower, 1966).

[9]As in *American Airlines*, Note 8 above. Also *Green River Steel Corp.*, 49 LA 117, 67–2 ARB ¶8469 (Chalfie, 1967), where the grievant had been previously warned about his drinking problem and the unexcused absences to which it led. His discharge was sustained after he was arrested and jailed for public drunkenness, failed to "report off" from work that day, and missed the next three days, claiming illness. *Eastern Air Lines, Inc.*, 45 LA 932 (Ables, 1965), presents similar facts.

In *Lamb Glass Co.*, 32 LA 420 (Dworkin, 1959), cited above, the arbitrator withheld back pay from the grievant, though his discharge in connection with a drunk driving arrest was overturned, in view of his inability to work as scheduled and to report his absence during his confinement in jail. (Discharge for those offenses was not warranted, since the grievant's absence did not significantly interfere with production schedules or the earnings of his crew.)

[10]Discharge was upheld, for example, in *Cities Service Oil Co.*, 41 LA 1091 (Oppenheim, 1963), where an employee who was involved in an automobile accident while driving under the influence of alcohol (an offense for which he was also arrested) missed nearly four months' work as a result.

[11]*Combustion Engineering, Inc.*, 80 LA 503 (Heinsz, 1983), where the grievant became drunk and rowdy in a tavern across the street from the plant, went outside, and threw empty beer bottles through the plant windows, causing over $600 damage; his discharge was sustained. In *Hydro-Electric Commission of Mississauga*, 68 LA 1230 (O'Shea, 1977), the grievant was found to be accountable for damaging a vehicle belonging to the employer when he stopped for a few drinks after work, then had an accident while driving the truck home; discharge was held to be too severe, however, since a supervisor had turned the truck over to him at the bar where both had been drinking, knowing that the grievant was not completely sober.

- Off-premises fighting or other conflict involving company personnel.[12]

Condition No. 3: The drinker has a company vehicle in his custody when he's drinking off the clock.

An employee who drinks while in charge of a company vehicle becomes subject to discipline even if no damage is done and even if he does not become intoxicated. An employee who is responsible for company property off the job is no different, with respect to his obligation to protect that property by remaining sober, from an employee whose on-the-job drinking might endanger company property on the premises.

> *Arbitrator Maslanka:* "Because the employee involved, B__, albeit on a non-paid lunch break was still in possession of City equipment and charged with its safe operation, I would liken this case to one in which the Employer promulgates and enforces reasonable rules while the employee is still on the Employer's premises.
>
> "There can be no question for example that an Employer operating an oil refinery could enforce a rule against smoking, even during non-paid lunch breaks. I find the rule in this case to have the same reasonable rationale—safety of fellow employees and the public in general."[13]

Condition No. 4: The drinker is a truck driver (or bus driver, etc.) who gets into trouble for mixing driving and drinking.

Most arbitrators would agree that employees who drive motor vehicles as part of their jobs are subject to discipline if they are convicted for driving under the influence or get involved in an accident while intoxicated.[14]

[12] *NCR, Appleton Papers Division, Locks Mill,* 70 LA 756 (Gundermann, 1978), where the grievant while under the influence vandalized a supervisor's home and automobile, and the arbitrator reasoned that his return to work would have a "negative impact on supervisory personnel thus affecting the Company's ability to direct the workforce."

[13] *City of Milwaukee,* 71 LA 329, 330 (Maslanka, 1978). See also: *General Tire Service,* 52 LA 1279, 69–2 ARB ¶8755 (Todd, 1969) (company rule prohibiting "drinking related to employment" covered situation in which employee was drinking while in possession of company truck that he took home in case of emergency call) and *Browning-Ferris Industries of Ohio, Inc., 77 LA 289 (Shanker, 1981)* (rule prohibitiing "drinking on duty" applied to lunchtime-drinking driver). Discipline was also justified in the case of three police officers who went drinking and "joy riding" in a patrol car, though discharge was ruled too severe since one of their supervisors was aware of their plans and let them take the car. (*City of Royal Oak,* 83–1 ARB ¶8254 (Howlett, 1983))

[14] On the differences between arrest, indictment and conviction for criminal offenses, see JUST CAUSE, Chapter 5.

Arbitrator Ludolf: "It is not unreasonable for an employer to consider the off duty drinking habits of one of its truck drivers as directly related to his employment driving habits. If he drives his own car while under the influence there is adequate reason to believe that he might do the same while on duty."[15]

In other words, what is called into question in this type of case is an employee-driver's reliability. The fact that a driver/employee runs afoul of drinking and driving laws while off duty does not *necessarily* mean he would do the same while on the job; but even the *possibility* that he might do so is serious enough to justify preventive measures.

Of course, if an employee loses his driver's license as a result of an off-clock incident, he loses an essential job qualification. In this situation, the employer may voluntarily put him in a nondriving job instead of terminating him (if the job assignment provisions of the contract so permit), but is not required to do so absent contract language requiring reassignment.[16]

Condition No. 5: The company has a rule covering alcohol use immediately before work or during breaks.

It's clear that if an employee stops for a couple of beers during his lunch break, discipline can follow if, as a result, he reports under the influence. But what happens if those couple of beers have no noticeable effect? Is it the employer's business?

SUPPOSE: *Where there's a rule, the company has a way.*

Helen Workman is suspended for 10 days for drinking a beer during the four-hour interval between the two parts of her split shift in violation of a company rule prohibiting the consumption of alcoholic

[15]*Angelica Corp.*, 62 LA 1227, 1229 (Bryan, 1974). Similarly, Arbitrator Ludolf: "Since the grievant was a truck driver, his driving record both on and off the job does seem to be relevant. Certainly, a worker with several charges of driving while intoxicated would not appear to be a good risk in a job that requires driving. While he had not yet been charged with drinking on the job or appearing for work in an intoxicated condition, there is also no evidence that his drinking problem had diminished. . . . While protecting the rights of an individual employee are [sic] important, such must not be at the expense of endangering innocent parties or the general public." (*Texas Automatic Sprinklers, Inc.*, 76–2 ARB ¶8493 (1976)) The grievant's discharge following a serious accident in which he was charged with driving under the influence was sustained.

In *Angelica Corp.*, the grievant was fired for having had three on-the-job accidents within a 45–day period and finally getting arrested for driving while intoxicated. Discharge was rescinded since not all the accidents were entirely his fault, but a 60–day suspension was imposed. In still another truck driver case, *Akers Motor Lines, Inc.*, 41 LA 987 (Woodruff, 1963), the grievant, who pleaded *nolo contendere* to a drunk driving charge, was reinstated without back pay in view of his long good record and the fact that he did not lose his license.

[16]*Texas Automatic Sprinklers, Inc.*, 76–2 ARB ¶8493 (Ludolf, 1976).

beverages at any time during an employee's tour of duty, including breaks. The union protests that Workman was not claimed to be under the influence when she reported back to work and that the company's policy is arbitrary and unreasonable.

Did the suspension stick? It did. Concluding that a company has a legitimate interest in preventing employees from coming to work after drinking, the arbitrator disagreed that Workman's off-clock drinking was none of the employer's business. While conceding that four hours is longer than the average break, he noted that the company had a strong emphasis on public relations. Moreover, Workman was well aware of the rule she violated, having signed a copy of it several months earlier, and the policy had been enforced uniformly and evenhandedly. Under those circumstances, 10 days off was not too harsh a penalty.[17]

In other words, "yes"—an employee may be penalized for having a drink or two before work or with his lunch—with a couple of "ifs."

First "if": Employees must be given advance notice that discipline will be imposed for having a drink during a break or within a certain number of hours before a shift. The same is true of rules that prohibit drinking when an employee is "on call" or "subject to duty" and may have to report to work on short notice.[18] As in *General Telephone,* a clearly promulgated rule normally satisfies that notice requirement.[19]

Second "if": The company must have a special need to protect itself against the possible adverse effects of break-time drinking by prohibiting such drinking entirely. In *General Telephone,* for example, "the Company's extensive contact with the public and, accordingly, its legitimate, even vital, stake in promoting positive employee–customer relations" made complete prohibition of drinking reasonable. And where

[17]*General Telephone Co. of California,* 77 LA 1052 (Schuster, 1981).

[18]E.g., *General Tire and Service Corp.,* 52 LA 1279, 69–2 ARB ¶8755 (Todd, 1969), where discharge was upheld in the case of an employee who was found drinking off company premises when he was "on call" for late evening emergencies and was in possession of a company vehicle. Also see cases cited by Denenberg and Denenberg, ALCOHOL AND DRUGS: Issues In The Workplace (Washington: BNA Books, (1983), pp. 117–18.

[19]Union acquiescence to such a rule (either by explicit agreement or by failure to protest the rule's existence) strengthens the company's right to penalize off-clock drinking still further, as illustrated by *International Pipe and Ceramics Corp.,* 44 LA 267, 65–1 ARB ¶8126 (Grant, 1965). Because it had for some time experienced problems with employees drinking at meal breaks, the company attached an "amendment" to its no-drinking rule to the effect that meal-break drinking could henceforth result in discharge. When an employee was terminated for violating that "amendment," the arbitrator rejected the union's argument that the company had no right to punish employees for off-premises activities unless they were unfit to work at reporting time. The union had led management to believe that it, too, saw an evil in lunch-hour drinking and that management's efforts to curtail it would have union support.

safety is of vital importance to an employer, as in the transportation industry, rules prohibiting all preshift or break-time drinking are common.

An employer's need to maintain a "sober" image for public relations purposes also normally justifies a rule of this type, the rationale being that customers who saw a company employee having a drink before work would have no way of knowing whether he would be sober when he reported to work and might lose confidence in the company.[20] Rules prohibiting drinking while in company uniform have been held to be reasonable for the same reason.[21]

> THE CONNECTION—In Re: Notice
>
> In this sensitive area where the employer seeks to interfere with employees' personal lives, notice of restrictions on off-premises conduct must be clearly and adequately communicated. The more indirect the connection between an employee's drinking and his job, the clearer the notice needs to be.[22]

[20]Rules prohibiting the use of alcoholic beverages by flight crews during the 12–hour (or even 24–hour) period before a flight are standard practice, for example, in the airline industry for *both* safety *and* image reasons. Arbitrator Turkus, in *Northwest Airlines, Inc.*, 1975 ARB ¶8207: "In my opinion, the drinking of any alcoholic beverage by a cockpit crew member in violation of the 24–hour rule is an egregious offense of such magnitude and gravity as to destroy that employee's further usefulness, value and entitlement to continued employment."

[21]As in *Eastern Greyhound Lines,* 70–2 ARB ¶8789 (Kelliher, 1970), upholding bus driver-grievants' suspensions for drinking beer at lunch in violation of a rule prohibiting drinking while wearing any part of a company uniform; or *Pacific Greyhound Lines,* 25 LA 709, 714–15 (Lennard, 1955), where the arbitrator noted: "Where services intimately affect the lives and safety of the public, it may well be that the appearance of fact is almost as important as the fact itself. . . . It is probably not only public alarm which the company seeks to avoid by its rule against drivers' drinking in uniform. Company officials are also entitled to be free from such alarm. They ought to be free from any doubt about whether a driver drank while driving or drank after he arrived at the depot."

[22]The rules involved in the cases discussed above were as follows:

N.Y.S. Dept of Correctional Services: "Every employee, whether on or off duty, shall so comport himself as to reflect credit on the department, the institution and its personnel. Any conduct constituting disorderly conduct or a misdemeanor or a felony within the meaning of the penal law may be the basis for disciplinary action whether or not prosecuted or a conviction results."

Polk County, Iowa: "Employees are expected to use good taste and judgment in their conversation, attitude, conduct and personal appearance to help maintain a good relationship with fellow employees and with the public. Disciplinary action may be taken against employees for . . . engaging in conduct considered to be incompatible with employment. . . ."

Lockheed Aircraft Corp: Discipline possible for "misconduct on company property or elsewhere, adversely affecting the interest or reputation of the Company or its employees."

Note, however: Even in cases where an off-clock drinking rule is clearly reasonable, alleged violations (like violations of any rule) must be *proved* before any penalty is imposed. The fact that off-clock, off-premises drinking may be difficult for an employer to police, and therefore to prove, does not reduce his burden in that respect. The possibility that an employee *may* have been drinking is not enough.[23]

Furthermore, as in any case, the penalty must be appropriate under all the circumstances. In one airlines case involving a rule barring drinking during the 24–hour period before a flight, for example, the arbitrator concluded that it was less serious for a flight attendant to have a glass of wine with dinner than it would have been for a pilot to do the same thing. In the absence of specific notice that any employee violating the rule would be terminated, discharge for a first offense was too harsh.[24]

Condition No. 6: The employer's public image is at stake.

Alcohol can get an employee into many kinds of trouble that the employer might justifiably argue can adversely affect his reputation and therefore his ability to conduct his business.

FOR EXAMPLE:

In *N.Y.S. Dept of Correctional Services,* 69 LA 345 (Kornblum, 1977), the arbitrator observed that the grievant's drinking and brawling in local bars "hardly reflected credit on the Department's or a Peace Officer's needful public image as an instrument and adjunct of law enforcement" (at 350); though extenuating circumstances were present that led the arbitrator to return the grievant to work (without back pay), he did so only on condition that the grievant relinquish his right to carry a firearm off duty.

[23]In *Western Air Lines, Inc.*, 37 LA 130 (Wyckoff, 1961), evidence that a flight attendant reported for duty tardy and in a disheveled condition was found insufficient to establish that she had been drinking, where company testimony that her breath smelled of alcohol was not convincing. (Suspension for tardiness and poor public appearance was justified, however, even if discharge for drinking was not.) Even where a bus driver was arrested for public drunkenness less than four hours before his next trip, discharge was not sustained where the arbitrator was not persuaded that the charges were valid. *Greyhound Lines-East,* 74–2 ARB ¶8385 (Kelliher, 1974).

[24]*Northwest Airlines, Inc.*, 56 LA 837, 71–1 ARB ¶8346 (Wyckoff, 1971). The arbitrator similarly found in *Trans World Airlines,* 38 LA 1221 (Wallen, 1962), that summary discharge was too severe for a flight attendant who admitted drinking a glass of champagne within 12 hours of her flight; while in *National Grocers Co., Ltd.*, 57 LA 637 (Weatherill, 1971), the discharge of a truck driver for lunchtime drinking was commuted to a reinstatement without back pay because the company had given other violators of the same rule lesser penalties.

Arrests for drunken driving often bring employees into collision with this type of rule, and in many cases discipline up to and including discharge has been upheld. In *Polk County Iowa,* 80 LA 639 (Madden, 1983), for example, the grievant, who worked as a counselor in a state correctional facility, pleaded guilty to a charge of driving under the influence—conduct which the employer and the arbitrator found to be incompatible with her responsibility to serve as a role model to her clients and to present a good image to the community. In *Lockheed Aircraft Corp.,* 37 LA 906 (T. Roberts, 1961), the arbitrator upheld the grievant's discharge after he had two alcohol-related auto accidents while on out-of-town assignment that brought the company adverse publicity.

The case of *Lamb Glass Co.,* 32 LA 420 (H. Dworkin, 1959) illustrates the problems that the company can run into. Although the company claimed to have had a long-established rule to the effect that an employee convicted of drunken driving would be subject to immediate discharge, the rule had never been reduced to writing or posted, and a conflict arose as to whether the grievant had been made aware of the rule when he was hired. Furthermore, the phrasing of the rule did not make it clear that it was intended to apply to off-duty driving as well as to driving on the job. The arbitrator's conclusion:

> "Since as a matter of 'common law' applicable to industrial relations, what an employee does on his own time is not a subject of regulation by the employer, any qualifying restriction must be expressly set out in clear and unequivocal language. In the absence of such language evidencing a contrary intent, it must be concluded that the language . . . was designed and intended to apply to employees during working hours." (at 423)

Since the business was not of an especially sensitive nature, so that employees should have known even without a rule that a drunk driving arrest might be of direct concern to the employer, the grievant's discharge was not upheld.

Condition No. 7: An employee has had previous difficulties because of chronic alcoholism, and his continued employment depends on his remaining strictly "on the wagon."

Notice is also at the heart of this final "condition" linking an employee's off-premises drinking with his job. In cases where an employee with a serious drinking problem is being retained on a "last chance" basis, one not-uncommon stipulation is that he keep away from alcohol entirely—on the job or off. If he violates that condition, discharge will normally follow.

> *Arbitrator Draper:* "Ordinarily management does not reserve a right to supervise an employee's personal life away from the plant, but where as here a condition has been placed on an employee's reinstatement to avoid a certain place [a local tavern frequented by employees at lunchtime] because of his weakness, which affects him, his disobedience of a plant rule, and the hazardous conditions of his employment, then such condition is valid."[25]

III. THE CASE OF THE CHRONIC ALCOHOLIC

The chronic alcoholic presents a special problem within the context of discharge for just cause—not simply the "drinking man" whose fondness for tying one on gets him into trouble periodically, but the individual whose physical and psychological dependency on alcohol constitutes an illness as defined by medical authorities.

WHAT IS A CHRONIC ALCOHOLIC? NINE CRITERIA

Arbitrator Ratner has set forth the following abbreviated *"Criteria for the Diagnosis of Alcoholism,"* which were compiled by a committee of medical authorities from the National Council on Alcoholism:

> "(1) *Physiological dependency* as evidenced by a withdrawal syndrome when the intake of alcohol is interrupted or decreased, i.e., gross tremors, withdrawal seizures, etc.
>
> "(2) *Evidence of tolerance* to the effects of alcohol as indicated by blood alcohol level of more than 150 mg without gross evidence of intoxication.
>
> "(3) *Symptom of a variety of major alcohol-associated illnesses:* alcoholic hepatitis, chronic gastritis, fatty degeneration in the absence of other known causes, etc.
>
> "(4) *Psychological dependence* on alcohol as evidenced by marriage disruption because of drinking, arrest for intoxication, driving while intoxicated, etc.

[25]*Sterling Drug, Inc.*, 67 LA 1296, 1300 (Draper, 1976). See also *Emge Packaging Co.*, 52 LA 195, 69–1 ARB ¶8417 (Uible, 1968), where the grievant was reinstated after a previous termination on the condition that he attend Alcoholics Anonymous and stop drinking completely. Discharge for drinking on his own time was sustained.

"(5) *Physiological and clinical effects* as noticed by odor of alcohol on breath, or vascular engorgement of face, or tachycardia or flushed face, etc.

"(6) *Behavioral effects* such as gulping drinks, surreptitious drinking, morning drinking, or indirect effects.

"(7) *Indirect behavioral effects* such as outbursts of rage and suicidal gestures.

"(8) *Psychological and attitudinal effects,* such as, when talking freely, making frequent references to drinking alcohol, people being 'bombed,' 'stoned,' or admits drinking more than peer group.

"(9) *Indirect effects* as evidenced by spouse making complaints about drinking behavior or major family disruptions or complaints about wife, job and friends." (*Monsanto Chemical Co.,* 79–2 ARB ¶8410 (1979)).

Alcoholism *per se* is generally not considered to be a basis for discharge or other discipline, any more than any other type of illness. Even if a supervisor believes that the chronic alcoholic is morally weak and therefore undesirable to have around, he needs to recognize that that attitude is no longer generally accepted and that, in the great majority of cases, an employee cannot be terminated solely because he is an alcoholic—*so long as* he manages to keep his drinking separate from his working life.[26]

If the problem comes to the employer's attention before drinking gets the employee into trouble on the job, some intervention may take place at that stage, since an increasing number of companies have recognized that alcoholism is an illness and provide employees with the *opportunity for rehabilitation*—for example, by granting medical leaves of absence for in-hospital treatment or using other accepted in-patient treatment methods.

Obviously, the first-line supervisor's responsibility at this stage will be defined by the particular employer's policies vis-à-vis alcoholism and its treatment. His role may be limited to keeping his eyes open to see if the employee who has been coming in later and later (for example) looks "hung over" or shows other predictable signs of a drinking problem. But the employer may not know that an employee suffers from alcoholism until some act of misconduct forces the problem to its attention. The employee may not even admit to himself that he has a

[26]For extended discussions of the full range of problems created by alcoholism in the work force and varying management approaches to the treatment of alcoholic employees, see books and articles cited in Appendix C.

problem; or with the help of family and friends—even his doctor—may try to hide it because he is ashamed, afraid of losing his job, or for other reasons.

Sympathetic first-line supervisors, too, have been known to cooperate in the cover-up, as the employee promises again and again to get his drinking under control.

ENTER THE QUESTION OF JUST CAUSE

But in most cases, an employee's alcoholism cannot be kept separate indefinitely from his working life, and his drinking problem finally surfaces in one of two kinds of employment-related misconduct that bring discipline into the picture:

Long-Term: Typically, a building pattern of absenteeism and/or tardiness finally reaches the point where the employer says, "Enough! We've walked that last mile with him!," and fires him.[27] Gradually declining productivity or work quality may also be involved.[28]

Short-Term: The employee's drinking finally explodes in some act of egregious misconduct. He shows up for work one morning "stewed to the gills," punches the supervisor who tries to send him home, and gets fired instead.[29]

As in those cases of off-premises drinking that cause an employee to violate some work rule (See Conditions 1 and 2 in Part II of this chapter), it is not the alcoholic's illness *per se* or even his drinking *per se* that is a potential basis for discipline but the misconduct to which

[27]See, e.g., *Indianapolis Rubber Co.*, 79 LA 529 (T. Gibson, 1982); *General Dynamics*, 79 LA 182 (Rule, 1982); *United States Steel Corp.*, 77 LA 855 (Hales, 1981); *General Abrasive Co.*, 81–2 ARB ¶8568 (Denson, 1981); *United States Steel Corp.*, 54 LA 760 (A. Wolff, 1970); *Active Products Co., 68–1 ARB ¶8103 (May, 1967); Eastern Air Lines, Inc.*, 45 LA 932 (Ables, 1965); *Caterpillar Tractor Co.*, 44 LA 87 (Larkin, 1965).

[28]As in *Green River Steel Corp.*, 49 LA 117, 69–2 ARB ¶8755 (Chalfie, 1967), in which there was a not-uncommon overall deterioration of the grievant's work habits. He appeared for work several times with alcohol on his breath; other employees lost respect for him and asked to be shifted so as not to work with him; he spent long periods in the men's room; his work performance became unsatisfactory; and he frequently had to ask other employees for help because he was physically unable to do his work. For a similar fact situation, see *Bethlehem Steel Corp.*, 54 LA 1090 (Porter, 1970).

[29]See *U.S. Steel Corp.*, 77 LA 854 (Hales, 1981) (grievant set out for work under influence of alcohol, drove speeding and recklessly into company parking lot, and cursed and resisted patrolman who chased and finally stopped him); *Lone Star Pennsuco, Inc.*, 80 LA 875 (Kanzer, 1983) (grievant reported for work intoxicated and caused accident resulting in considerable waste of company product); *Asarco, Inc.*, 76 LA 163 (Grooms, 1981) (grievant reported for work drunk); *NCR, Appleton Papers Division, Locks Mill*, 70 LA 756 (Gundermann, 1978) (grievant got drunk off premises and vandalized supervisor's home and car); *Park Haven Care Center*, 79–2 ARB ¶8328 (Fitzsimmons, 1979).

alcohol abuse leads. For most employees, any of the examples of long-term and short-term misconduct cited above would be a reasonable basis for discharge or other form of discipline. But the question that remains is whether in the special case of the alcoholic, his illness absolves him of responsibility for his behavior so that he is not subject to discipline in the same manner as other employees. The case could be made, as one arbitrator has put it, that misconduct "occurred not because of an indifference toward the Company rules but because he was emotionally and physically sick."[30] Or to put this proposition another way—where there is no *intention* to commit misconduct, misconduct as such does not exist. Rehabilitation efforts may be called for—but not discharge or other disciplinary penalty.

By and large, arbitrators have been willing to take the particular problems of the alcoholic employee into account in deciding whether just cause for discipline is present. Arbitrator Kesselman has set forth the prevailing philosophy concerning the employee whose alcohol problems first emerge through some form of misconduct:

> "It is now generally conceded that chronic alcoholism must be distinguished from normal drinking habits. The alcoholic person has come to be regarded by medical experts as suffering from a disease which causes him to become a compulsive drinker in contrast with a normal person who can control his intake of alcohol.
>
> "Because of this knowledge, it is now customary in American industry to view alcoholism with sympathetic understanding as an illness rather than as a mortal sin.
>
> "Rather than summarily imposing disciplinary penalties upon employees suffering from chronic alcoholism, as the Union points out, it has become increasingly common for companies to encourage such employees to recognize that they have a drinking problem and to seek treatment for it and to provide assistance through leaves of absence, payment of treatment costs, sick pay benefits during treatment, etc."[31]

But no arbitrator would go so far as to say that because an employee suffers from alcoholism, the company can never terminate his employment.

[30] *Armstrong Cork Co.*, 56 LA 527, 529, 71–1 ARB ¶8242 (B. Wolf, 1971).

[31] *American Synthetic Rubber Corp.*, 73–1 ARB ¶8070 (1973).

> *Arbitrator J. Duff:* "The state of being under the influence of alcohol, even where it may be an involuntary incident of alcoholism, is not as such a legitimate excuse for absenteeism or a condition which somehow relieves an employee of responsibility for failing to be present at work. . . . The Company is correct in its assertion that as a general policy it need not accept alcoholism as a disease that totally obscures individual responsibility for absenteeism."[32]

The overriding question, then, involves a balancing of interests—on the one hand, there is the employer's responsibility to help the alcoholic employee, and on the other, there is the right to terminate any employee who cannot do his job. (Some would say that different balances must be struck in the private and public sectors; in the private sector the employer would be required to go "the last mile," whereas in the public sector the employer would be required to go "the last mile and one-half" before terminating the employee.) The question of balancing these two interests is explored further in Chapter 7, PENALTY.

[32]*Damascus Steel Casting Co.,* 80–1 ARB ¶8188, 3857 (J. Duff, 1980). To the same effect, Arbitrator Lewis: "Successful defenses have been raised in criminal prosecutions involving specific intent because of alcohol or drug content, the cases holding that a man under the influence of alcohol cannot be guilty of an intentional act. It must not be assumed, however, that because the grievant's actions may not have been intended, they did not have any standing or were nonexistent. The grievant's conduct, whether intended or not, did not conform to the minimum standards necessary to maintain work status." (*Koppers, Inc.,* 79–2 ARB ¶8613, 5742 (1979))

Arguments that the alcoholic grievant should be forgiven because he was not responsible for his actions, or could not control his behavior, have also been rejected in *Standard Packaging Corp.,* 71 LA 445 (Fogelberg, 1978); *Bi-State Development Agency,* 76 LA 1178 (Rohlik, 1981); and *General Abrasive Co.,* 81–2 ARB ¶8568 (Denson, 1981).

Chapter 3

INVESTIGATION

"Did the employer, *before* administering the discipline to an employee, make an effort to discover whether the employee did in fact violate or disobey a rule or order of management?"

INTRODUCTION

Arbitrator Gentile: " 'Just cause' is a multi-faceted consideration which has been applied by Arbitrators to fact portraits in various ways. A thread which runs through these numerous decisions is the concept that the Company make a *full, fair and objective investigation* in order to be satisfied that the charged individual is in fact guilty of the offense or breach"[1] (emphasis added).

Whenever discipline for any reason is contemplated, a timely, thorough investigation of suspected misconduct is critical to management for two reasons: first, as one of the more fundamental Daugherty tests, and also because it can have a domino effect upon two of the other tests.

First—sufficient proof: If management fails to make diligent efforts to uncover all the relevant facts and circumstances surrounding a suspected offense, it may easily end up without enough evidence to prove that any misconduct was actually committed—that is to say, failure on the "Investigation" test can lead to failure on the "Proof" test as well. And obviously, where no misconduct is established, no penalty at all can be justified.

[1]*Dow Chemical Co.*, 60 LA 703, 706–707 (1973).

Second—fair play: Due process requires that an employee (1) be informed promptly and with reasonable precision what offense he is being charged with, *and* (2) be given a fair opportunity to tell his own side of the story. If management takes disciplinary action without first getting *all* the available evidence—evidence in the employee's favor as well as evidence against him—the penalty may be overturned or reduced by an arbitrator because of that procedural violation alone, even if the evidence otherwise establishes that the employee is guilty.

The "Investigation" test is often of critical importance in the case of alcohol-related misconduct because the threshhold dispute in a large proportion of alcohol cases is whether the grievant in fact committed the offense—intoxication, drinking, or possession of alcohol. The basic criteria for an adequate investigation into any of these three types of misconduct are the same criteria required in disciplinary investigations in general, namely:

1. *All potential witnesses have been questioned.* That includes statements about the employee's actions and, in some cases, his physical condition, not only by members of management but also by the accused employee himself and any witnesses on his behalf.

2. *All relevant physical and documentary evidence has been obtained.* In alcohol cases, physical evidence typically means such evidence of drinking as liquor or beer bottles, while documentary evidence means the employee's work record, including any history of alcohol problems. Medical evidence, very important in many intoxication cases, also falls is documentary.

3. *The investigation has been pursued in a timely manner.* For the most part, investigation in alcohol cases is a routine matter. Chapter 5, which deals with the "Proof" test, sets forth in detail what constitutes proof of the three different types of alcohol-related misconduct—and in doing so, tells the supervisor what specific kinds of evidence his investigation normally needs to cover in each type of case. This chapter focuses on three areas of alcohol investigation which often raise special problems.

A PREVIEW

Three special issues in Investigation:

I. Blood Alcohol Tests
- Must an employer use these tests?
- May an employee say, "No thanks"?
- A two-way street

II. The "Search and Seizure" Issue

III. Time is of the Essence
- In re: Proof
- In re: Due Process

I. BLOOD ALCOHOL TESTS

MUST AN EMPLOYER USE THESE TESTS?

The Rule

In many cases where an employee is charged with being under the influence of alcohol, the union argues that even the most thorough evaluation of his behavior and appearance is not enough to prove intoxication. To be conclusive and complete, according to this view, the company's investigation must also include the results of a blood alcohol test (commonly known as a "sobriety test") in which a blood, urine, or breath sample is taken from an individual and then analyzed to determine the level of alcohol in his bloodstream.

Most arbitrators, however, do not place alcohol tests on that kind of pedestal. Supervisors, they say, are competent to decide whether an employee is under the influence on the sole basis of their own observations of an employee's behavior.[2] A blood alcohol test may be desirable by way of corroboration, but only in the exceptional case has an

[2]"Proving that one is under the influence of an intoxicant does not necessarily require that there be a blood test. . . . A test might bolster the Company's case or it might not. In any event, this is the Company's decision, and if it chooses to take action on the basis of testimony of witnesses it can do so without being faulted." (*Golden Foundry, Inc.*, 76–1 ARB 8012, 4557 (Traynor, 1975). To similar effect: *Hunt Foods and Industries, Inc.*, 64–3 ARB 8960, 6318 (Hebert, 1964) ("being under the influence of liquor, as applied to plant operations, does not depend upon an ability to prove with scientific accuracy and by sobriety tests that an employee has overindulged"); *Peoples Gas Light & Coke Co.*, 74–2 ARB ¶8552 (P. Davis, 1974); *The Taylor-Winfield Corp.*, 66–2 ARB ¶8406 (Stouffer, 1966).

arbitrator been so skeptical about the reliability of direct evidence that he required the company to produce blood alcohol test results.[3] (For a detailed discussion of the relative strengths and weaknesses of direct evidence and blood alcohol test evidence, see Chapter 5, beginning at p. 56).

The Exceptions

There are *three situations* in which a blood alcohol test may have to be part of an investigation of intoxication.

1. *Where the employee requests the opportunity to be tested.* An employee's request for a sobriety test places the whole "to test or not to test" question in a different framework. A desire to be tested on the suspected employee's part strongly suggests that he is confident of his innocence and may tip the weight of the evidence in his favor, especially where the direct evidence against him is less than overwhelming. Under these circumstances, the company's failure to arrange to have him tested may be interpreted as denying him a reasonable opportunity to defend himself—a breach of his due process rights.

FOR EXAMPLE:

That Workman asked for and was denied a test was "most impressive" to the arbitrator, where his symptoms were compatible with lingering effects of alcohol from a previous night's drinking, and where he carried out his duties without any noticeable problem.[4]

2. *Where the employee raises one of the "Three Classic Defenses" against intoxication charges: "It's my medication!"—"I'm sick!"—"It's those fumes!"* In some cases, many typical symptoms of intoxication—poor physical coordination, a "stuporous" appearance, slurred speech, etc.—can be produced by something other than excessive drinking. Where an employee protests that he was really "under the influence" of medication or something other than alcohol, a blood

[3]E.g., *Northrop Worldwide Service, Inc.*, 64 LA 742 (Goodstein, 1975), where the arbitrator acknowledged frankly that his refusal to rely exclusively on supervisors' judgments represented a minority position.

[4]*Park Haven Care Center, Inc.*, 79–2 ARB ¶8328 (Fitzsimmons, 1979). A similar conclusion was reached in *Continental Conveyor & Equipment Co.*, 69 LA 1143, 77–2 ARB ¶8598 (Tucker, 1977), where the grievant's request for a sobriety test weighed more heavily with the arbitrator than his (playful) statement to the foreman which triggered his discharge: "I'm drunk again."

alcohol test may offer the company a reasonably definitive opportunity (perhaps its only opportunity) to send his explanation packing.

3. *In any case where direct evidence that an employee is under the influence has any significant flaws.*

MAY AN EMPLOYEE SAY, "NO THANKS"?

Suppose the company decides to play it safe and arranges for an employee who is suspected of having had one too many to take a sobriety test at a local hospital or clinic. Have union complaints about "unfair investigation" been headed off at the pass? Not necessarily. The company may now find itself facing an altogether different argument from the union, namely, that the company has no right to insist that an employee submit to a blood alcohol test if he chooses not to take one.

Taking the "Fifth"

The contention that an employee may say "No, thanks" to a blood test, without having the refusal counted against him in any way, flows from the proposition that the constitutional privilege against self-incrimination guaranteed to individuals as citizens under the Fifth Amendment carries over into the workplace and applies to them *as employees.* Arguments for and against that proposition are discussed at length in the volume on *Proof.* The "majority" position on this issue is summed up as follows by one of the leading adherents of that position, Arbitrator Meltzer:

> "The Union's contention raises the question of whether the privilege operates in an arbitration proceeding to bar evidence of a grievant's refusal to take an intoxication test when the only purpose and effect of that evidence relates to the propriety of Company discipline. For the reasons that follow, *this arbitrator answers 'No' to that question.*
>
> "The privilege against self-incrimination operates to protect individuals in their relations with government, and, specifically, is designed to provide protection against the risk of criminal penalties arising from compulsion of government. See McCormick, Evidence 268 (1954). The relationship between an employer and his employees is significantly different from the relationship between a state and its citizens. . . . The

penalties imposed by the state for criminal offenses are also materially different from discharge by the employer, despite the seriousness of discharge in some situations."[5]

What Then Does a Refusal to Be Tested Mean?

Some collective bargaining agreements (notably in transportation and other industries where employee sobriety is crucial for safety reasons) provide explicitly that an employee who is suspected of being intoxicated will be required to take a blood alcohol test, and a refusal to do so will be considered as an admission of guilt. But even where the contract or company rules are silent on a blood alcohol test requirement, most arbitrators will draw an *adverse inference* from any employee's refusal to be tested—meaning (in plain English) that if an employee balks at being tested, it logically means that he knows he is drunk and does not want that fact objectively confirmed.[6]

An exception to that general rule occurs where an employee can provide a satisfactory reason for his reluctance to take a test, and is not just afraid he will not "pass." One employee's explanation that he was afraid the plant manager was "out to get" him was accepted by the arbitrator—not as truth but as the employee's sincere belief.

SUPPOSE: *Grounds for suspicion*

When Harry Workman is accused of ramming his truck into a loading dock belonging to one of the employer's customers, he understandably gets upset and excited. On that evidence, the customer decides Harry must be drunk and calls Workman's employer. As a result, several supervisors speed to the scene and demand that Workman take a sobriety test. Workman refuses and is discharged.

[5]*Maremont Corp.* (Meltzer, 1969) (emphasis added); unpublished opinion quoted in Fairweather, Practice and Procedure in Labor Arbitration (Washington, D.C.: BNA, 1973), p. 251. See also *Tennessee River Pulp & Paper Co.,* 68 LA 421 (Simon, 1976) (blood test requirement not a violation of Fifth, Fourth, or Fourteenth Amendment); *New York Telephone Co.,* 66 LA 1037, 76–2 ARB ¶8420 (Markowitz, 1976) (results of blood test taken while grievant was unconscious in hospital admissible); *Bi-State Development Agency,* 72 LA 198 (Newmark, 1979) ("since this is not a criminal matter . . . the question of constitutional right is not involved"). *Capital Area Transit Authority,* 69 LA 811, 815 (Ellman, 1977), which holds that "a waiver of constitutional rights cannot be presumed," represents a minority position.

[6]As in *Hughes Air Corp.,* 76–1 ARB ¶8169, 5250 (Wyckoff, 1976) (refusal to take sobriety test justified conclusion that employee was intoxicated); and in *Kaiser Sand & Gravel,* 49 LA 190 (Koven, 1967), where the arbitrator found that the grievant's attempt to delay taking a sobriety test was "more that of a person who was hoping to prove that he was not drunk than it was the conduct of a person who was trying to prove that he had not been drinking at all. . . ." See KEY CASES IN DETAIL.

"Adverse inference" justified? Not in this case. The allegation that Workman was under the influence was extremely far-fetched, the arbitrator found. His only "symptom" was his excited manner, and even company witnesses admitted that he often spoke rapidly and incoherently when upset. Workman's explanation that he was afraid to take a blood test only because he thought the company was planning to "set him up" therefore rang true to the arbitrator. Even if the company had no such intention, the way in which company personnel overreacted to the customer's complaint gave Workman reason to be suspicious.

No adverse inference—no proof of intoxication—no discharge.[7]

Another exception: Lack of notice that a sobriety test may be required has also led arbitrators to decide that an employee's refusal to be tested should not be held against him;[8] arbitrators and the NLRB, however, both have held that an employee cannot justify refusing to take a blood alcohol test solely on the ground that a union representative is not present.[9]

A TWO-WAY STREET

The following observations by Arbitrator Sass help put in perspective the whole question of what place blood alcohol tests occupy in an investigation of intoxication:

First, from the company's standpoint: "The Company is not obligated to have blood test evidence to support its case. Such evidence

[7]*Blue Diamond Co.,* 66 LA 1136 (Summers, 1976). In *Consolidation Coal Co.,* 82–2 ARB ¶8605, 5706 (Sass, 1982), the arbitrator found, "Certainly an adverse inference might be drawn against a Grievant who refuses to have [a blood test] done when it is offered to him at or close to the Company premises. . . . But the fact that there was a severe rainstorm in progress and the nearest place he knew to be tested was 60 miles away over two lane country roads prevents the Arbitrator from making any significant conclusions from the Grievant's failure to get a blood test in this case." In *Bi-State Development Agency,* 72 LA 198 (Newmark, 1979), the Arbitrator did not sustain the discharge of a grievant who refused a sobriety test that he believed was biased in the company's favor; he offered, however, to take a test at another clinic.

[8]See Chapter 1, "Notice," p. 8.

[9]In *Bethlehem Steel Corp.,* 55 LA 994 (1955), Arbitrator Seward based his conclusion that the grievant was obliged to take a breathalyzer test, despite the company's denial of his request that a shop steward be present, on the theory that no question of disciplinary action had yet been raised at the time the grievant was given the choice of taking the tset or going home; "[h]e was being given an opportunity by a Plant Patrol officer to prove by a breathalyzer test that he was not under the influence of alcohol and was fit to enter the plant and go to work" (at 995). It is as yet unclear whether the Supreme Court's *Weingarten* decision (420 U.S. 251 (1975), which affirmed and solidified employees' rights to union representation during interviews which may even potentially lead to discipline, will have a significant effect in cases like *Bethlehem;* see *City of Milwaukee,* 78 LA 89 (Yaffe, 1982), for a recent statement of the problem.

would obviously be helpful and the Company takes a chance that, without such evidence, it will not be able to sustain its burden of proof. But the Company may go forward without it if it thinks it has a strong enough case."

Second, from the employee's standpoint: "Likewise, the Grievant is not obligated to get a blood alcohol test to prove his innocence. But the Grievant takes the chance that the Company's evidence will be strong enough to sustain the discharge unless he has something, such as favorable blood test results, to counteract the Company's case."[10]

A Gamble on Remedy

The grievant also takes the chance that even if the evidence ultimately falls short of proving that he was intoxicated and the arbitrator concludes that his discharge was not for just cause, his *remedy* may fall short if he has rejected the chance to clear himself by means of a sobriety test. As has been said and said again, in disciplinary matters the employer has the burden of proving his charges of misconduct and the employee is not obliged to disprove them. One might say that each is on his own. But when we come to the subject of investigation, there is a difference—each is not on his own; investigation is more of a two-way street and certain obligations to the other flow from that proposition.

The employer would have a frustrating time trying to determine all the facts and circumstances surrounding alleged misconduct, as the "Investigation" tests require, unless the employee cooperates by providing whatever evidence he can that works in his favor. If he refuses to cooperate, e.g., by not agreeing to take a blood alcohol test, most arbitrators will withhold back pay, even if he is ultimately cleared of intoxication charges. Usually the rationale is that he—and not the company—was responsible for the delay in resolving the dispute and he—not the company—must therefore pay the price.[11]

[10]*Consolidation Coal Co.,* 82–2 ARB ¶8605, 5705–6 (Sass, 1982).

[11]To award back pay, one arbitrator has noted, ". . . would largely frustrate some of the most important purposes of the sobriety test provision. The employee, by refusing to take the test, could prevent a quick and definitive determination of the issue on intoxication. Then in the arbitration proceedings . . . the employer will then have the heavy burden of proving intoxication by clear and convincing evidence, and with some arbitrators, beyond a reasonable doubt. In many intoxication cases evidence of such weight and clarity are difficult, if not impossible to obtain. . . . When one of the foremost purposes of the sobriety test provision is to provide a method for quick and definitive resolution of the intoxication issue, an employee who defeats that purpose by refusing to take that test ought not to be able to collect back pay during the delay which he himself has caused." (Blue Diamond Co., 66 LA 1136, 1142 (Summers, 1976))

II. SEARCH AND SEIZURE

REENTER THE CONSTITUTION

"Constitutional rights" issues may arise when an employer seeks to search an employee's person or belongings for liquor bottles or other tangible evidence of misconduct. Fourth Amendment safeguards against illegal search and seizure are sometimes invoked by an employee to justify his refusal to "open up" a locker, purse, lunch box, etc. But, as with Fifth Amendment protections against self-incrimination, most arbitrators agree that these constitutional rights do not apply in the strict sense in the industrial setting. An employee's refusal to consent to a search, therefore, may be accepted as evidence that he committed the suspected misconduct or may itself be ground for discipline for "lack of cooperation"—or both.[12]

SUPPOSE: *"Citizen v. employee"*

Miles Foreman sees Harry Workman take a drink "from a flat glass bottle containing an amber liquid." As he heads towards Workman, Workman turns his back, fumbling with his sweater. By the time Foreman reaches him, the sweater, which had previously been open, is buttoned securely. Workman refuses to "open up," standing on his constitutional rights, and denies ever having had a bottle in his possession. Nonetheless, the company suspends him for 15 days on two counts: having alcohol in his possession, and refusing to obey a supervisor's instructions.

Was the suspension justified? The arbitrator rejected Workman's "constitutional" defense with the observation:

"It is quite inappropriate to attempt to establish an exact parallel between rights of citizens on the street and employees in the plant. . . .

"If Grievant's view was adopted, an employee could steal valuable parts and secret them on his person and refuse to obey an order to disclose what he had on his person and thus avoid *any penalty* while the individual who admits his guilt or is caught in the process is discharged.

[12]The exceptional position, that "an employee does not lose the basic constitutional rights which a citizen enjoys, merely because the employee is exercising those rights within an industrial context," is represented by *Abex Corp.*, 79–2 ARB ¶8614 (Fitzgerald, 1979), where the arbitrator found that an employee could not be disciplined for refusing to open a package which appeared to contain a 12–pack of beer."[T]he existence of a right," he stated, "necessarily requires the ability to exercise that right without punishment. Therefore, the grievant's exercise of his right to refuse to have his personal property examined by the foreman was one for which he could not be disciplined. If discipline were to be allowed for the exercise of the right, then the right would effectively be denied to the person so exercising it" (at 5747).

The same is true of use of intoxicants, or drugs, the rule contended for puts a premium on stealth and lack of candor coupled with reliance on an inappropriate claim of constitutional privilege."

The company's dual grounds for suspending Workman thus held up: Foreman's order that Workman unbutton his sweater was reasonable, making Workman's refusal to comply an act of insubordination; furthermore, that refusal, coupled with Foreman's credible testimony that he had seen Workman drinking, amounted to convincing evidence that Workman had also violated the no-alcohol rule.[13]

EMPLOYEE RIGHTS: A DIFFERENT FRAMEWORK

In stressing the fact that the supervisor in the above case had "probable cause" to direct the grievant to open up, the arbitrator indirectly highlighted an important principle about "search and seizure" at the workplace: Those arbitrators who preclude employees from Fourth Amendment protection hold that employees are entitled to what might be called an "industrial version" of due process; an employer must, at the very least, show *some justifiable reason* (i.e., "probable cause") to order an employee to submit to a search (e.g., a supervisor's credible charge that he witnessed an act of misconduct). The requirement of "probable cause" might also be satisfied by a *prima facie* showing that a general problem with alcohol abuse had arisen on company premises that clearly called for preventive action.[14]

Prior notice may be required (as in the case of blood test requirements) if employees are to be directed to submit to a search or become subject to discipline. Such notice may take the form of negotiated contract language, a posted company rule, or even an established practice.[15]

[13]*Champion Spark Plug,* 68 LA 702, 705–706, 77–1 ARB ¶8158 (Casselman, 1977). A "split decision" was reached under similar facts in *Comco Metal Products, Ltd.,* 58 LA 279, 281 (H. Brown, 1972). The arbitrator, deciding that "there is no absolute right of an employer to search personal effects," found that the grievant's refusal to reveal the contents could not be used as evidence that she had alcohol in her possession, and her discharge for that offense could not be upheld. Her refusal was insubordinate, however, justifying the lesser penalty of a suspension.

[14]As in *Fruehauf Corp.,* 49 LA 89 (Daugherty, 1967), upholding the company's right to search lunch boxes for liquor in the face of a continuing problem with employees bringing intoxicants on company premises.

[15]In *Abex Corp.,* 79–2 ARB ¶8614 (Fitzgerald, 1979), the arbitrator found that *only* through company-union negotiations could a procedure for searching employees' personal property be established; but unilateral notice by the company of search requirements has been approved in other cases, e.g., *International Harvester Co.,* 77–1 ARB ¶8232 (Yarowsky, 1977).

III. TIME IS OF THE ESSENCE

IN RE: PROBLEMS OF PROOF

It is a commonplace to observe that investigation into employee misconduct should get under way as soon as practicable. But with alcohol-related situations it is even more important to move forward with dispatch as soon as any violation is suspected. Why? Because the evidence that is often required to prove possession, drinking, or intoxication has a tendency to disappear in a puff of smoke if the company does not move quickly.

IN THE MATTER OF "POSSESSION"— BEER? OR BOWLING SHOES?

Three employees are observed by management personnel carrying paper bags from the parking lot around to the back of the plant and depositing the bags in a weeded area. The employees enter the plant by the back door, whereupon the supervisors check the bags and find several six-packs of beer. Later that afternoon the employees are called in and charged with trying to bring alcohol into the plant. No such thing, they protest. They were carrying bags in the parking lot, sure—but the bags contained only bowling clothes and they carried them on into the plant. Other employees back them up, stating that they saw them inside with the bags.

The effect of the delay: An opportunity to prove what really happened was irretrievably gone.

"Why," the arbitrator asked, "didn't [A.] or one of the other officials call out to the men after they left the weeded area and headed for the plant door?" And why weren't the grievants confronted and asked about the bags as soon as they walked inside? "Whether or not they had bags (of beer? of bowling clothes and cigarettes?) with them before and/or after they entered the plant *would not now be one of the subjects of contradictory testimony.*" The company's proof thus fell flat.[16]

IN THE MATTER OF "DRINKING"—COVERING THE TRACES

Miles Foreman watches as Harry Workman lifts a whiskey bottle to his lips, then tosses the "empty" in a trash can. By the time Foreman can get to the scene, Workman is disappearing out another door, headed for lunch.

Foreman recovers the bottle and after lunch calls Workman into his office. Drinking? Absolutely not, says Workman.

[16]*Okonite Co.*, 74–2 ARB ¶8525, 4951 (Ludlow, 1974).

If Foreman had confronted Workman immediately after finding the whiskey bottle, he would have had a good chance of catching the odor of alcohol on his breath. An hour later, any alcohol smell had been wiped out by the food Workman had eaten. The company's evidence thus failed.[17]

IN THE MATTER OF "INTOXICATION"—
HERE TODAY, GONE TOMORROW

Harry Workman is having conspicuous difficulty keeping up with the production lines late one night; he sways and slumps on the seat of his forklift and fails to answer when spoken to, and another employee notices a smell of beer. Finally, Lem Bolton is called to the plant. He takes a look, tells Workman that he, too, smells beer, and walks away, leaving Workman to finish out the shift.

The next day the company asks Workman if he was intoxicated. He says no, but is discharged a few days later for working under the influence of alcohol.[18]

Two Problems of Proof—for the Price of One

The "delayed reaction" problem: If a supervisor fails to investigate promptly when intoxication is suspected, his "Oh, well. Let's wait and see" attitude may later be interpreted to mean that the employee's condition could not have been really serious. After all, what responsible supervisor would let an employee continue working if he believed he was unfit to do his job? (For several examples of this problem, see Chapter 5, p. 61.)

The disappearing act: Moreover, because the strongest symptoms of intoxication vanish with time as the body metabolizes the alcohol, the employer may forfeit all chance of proving that an employee is under the influence if he waits too long before giving the employee's condition a thorough appraisal.

> *Arbitrator Sembower:* "If he [the supervisor] thought the Grievant was in fact drunk rather than sick, it was incumbent upon him to stick to it. This is not a theoretical distinction, for one effect of his not doing so was to foreclose the parties from further exploring the question

[17]*St. Louis Diecasting Corp.*, 69–1 ARB ¶8163 (Erbs, 1968).

[18]*Merchants Refrigerating Co.*, unpublished opinion (Koven, 1983).

of drunkenness while the pros and cons then being actively disputed at a stage envisaged by the grievance procedure in the contract, could best be ascertained from 'live evidence.' "[19]

Take the case of the somnolent forklift driver, for example. Workman claimed at a later grievance hearing that he was in a stuporous condition that night because the medication that he was taking for a sinus headache "didn't agree with him" on top of a beer he had had before coming to work.

If Bolton had told Workman on the spot, "Harry, I believe you're drunk," and Workman had responded, "Hell, no—it's these sinus pills I'm taking," Bolton might have settled the matter right then and there by directing Workman to take a sobriety test. Instead, he walked away—and Workman went home to "sleep off" whatever evidence there might have been.

IN RE: DUE PROCESS

The Right to an Adequate Defense

Among an employee's basic rights which carry over from the criminal law to the industrial setting is the right to be told specifically, and in a timely manner, what misconduct he is being charged with. In the words of Arbitrator Seward:

> "An employee who does not know of what he is accused can obviously not defend himself against the accusation. If he is to have a 'reasonable opportunity' to present evidence in his behalf, he must be given at least some idea of the acts, event or issues to which his evidence—if it is to be relevant and persuasive—should relate."[20]

Under most circumstances, it is sufficient that the employer confront the grievant (and the union) with his accusations and provide a reasonable opportunity for the employee's response *at some point* before the employer reaches his final decision concerning discipline.

[19]*Hi-Life Packing Co.*, 41 LA 1083, 1086 (Sembower, 1963). Similarly, *Connor Mfg. Co.*, 63 LA 1102, 1105 (Mulhall, 1974): "While there are many occurrences where the situation is non-critical and where the events are such that good management requires a time for reflection and a period for discussion prior to taking final action, allegations of intoxication require immediate action."

[20]*Bethlehem Steel Co.*, 29 LA 635, 640 (1957).

Intoxication is a special case: Where intoxication is in issue, the timing of the employer's charges and investigation is more critical. For the same reason that a delayed investigation may result in problems of proof for the employer, the employee may likewise lose an essential opportunity to present evidence of his sobriety at the time his innocence can be most convincingly established.

Thus, to wrap up the case of the maybe-drunk/maybe-sick fork-lift driver, the supervisor, by failing to tell the grievant up front and right away that he was suspected of being intoxicated and that his job was in jeopardy, foreclosed the possibility that the grievant might volunteer to take a sobriety test or that he might seek a doctor's confirmation that he was sick. The grievant's ability to defend himself was compromised.

It could be argued that the grievant should have guessed from the supervisor's statement that he smelled beer that "prosecution" was a possibility. However, responsibility for observing due process rests with the company, and it would be unfair to transfer that burden to the employee, forcing him to guess when he is in jeopardy or what the charges are.[21]

[21]In *U.S. Steel Corp.*, 55 LA 677 (Wolff, 1979), the company initially charged the grievant with being in an unfit condition to work, but did not allege that intoxication was the reason until the arbitration hearing. Evidence of intoxication presented at the hearing, e.g., that a foreman smelled alcohol on his breath, came too late for the grievant to respond adequately to the charges; discharge was overturned.

Chapter 4

FAIR INVESTIGATION

"Was the Employer's investigation conducted fairly and objectively?"

A BIG POINT IN A SMALL PACKAGE

> " 'I'll be judge, I'll be jury,' said cunning old Fury; 'I'll try the whole cause, and condemn you to death.' "[1]

Daugherty's fourth just-cause test makes only a single point, but an important one. What it adds up to is this:

- For an investigation to be successful (from the point of view of both proof and due process) it must be objective;
- For it to be objective, someone from management must make certain that the evidence that has been collected is evaluated carefully, not just from a partisan, management-oriented perspective but from the perspective of a disinterested third party;
- Finally, the best person to conduct a disinterested evaluation and to make the final decision about disciplinary action ordinarily is some higher, detached management official and *not* the supervisor who was responsible for initiating disciplinary action.[2]

[1]Lewis Carroll, *Alice's Adventures in Wonderland*, Ch. 3.

[2]Daugherty explained what he had in mind in the notes to Question IV in these words: "Note 1: At said investigation, the management official may be both 'prosecutor' and 'judge' but he may not also be a witness against the employee. Note 2: It is essential for some higher, detached management official to assume and conscientiously perform the judicial role, giving the commonly accepted meaning to that term in his attitude and conduct. Note 3: In some disputes between an employee and a management person there are no witnesses to an incident other than the two immediate participants. In such cases, it is particularly important that the management 'judge' question the management participant rigorously and thoroughly, just as an actual third party would."

The thrust of this requirement: The supervisor who is an employee's principal accuser, or any supervisor who has produced evidence against him, has a natural tendency to believe that his view of what took place is accurate. Yet a supervisor, like anyone else, can always misperceive or misjudge a situation even in the best of faith. A supervisor may also have a hard time admitting that he was wrong if investigation turns up evidence that tends to support the grievant's side of the story.

For that reason, "fair investigation" requires that another company official step in and play the role of "judge," questioning management witnesses as thoroughly and critically as if he were a neutral third party; and that he make a decision on the facts, rather than automatically "backing up" his supervisor.

> *Arbitrator P. Seitz:* "Not infrequently, an employee is discharged because a supervisor has used bad judgment or because a personnel decision was made in haste or in the heat of controversy.
>
> "Tribal loyalty then encourages the employer to support a questionable initial decision through the grievance steps and in arbitration, even though second thoughts, more careful consideration, and later developed facts indicate that disciplinary suspension would be more just, fair, and consonant with the pattern of discipline in the plant."[3]

SUPPOSE:

Garage supervisor Lem Bolton is advised by Miles Foreman that in his judgment Harry Workman has been drinking. Workman, he says, called him over to the hoist where he was working and spoke to him about some transmission work in a loud and irrational manner; he also smelled of alcohol. Bolton tells Foreman, "Do what you have to do," and Foreman fires Workman.

An adequate reaction? No, according to the arbitrator.

"As manager of the garage operation, [Bolton] had the authority to countermand any decision of [Foreman], or urge him to seek additional confirmation of his suspicions before terminating [Workman] if he himself had any doubt whatever as to the propriety of such action. Instead, he *took no such steps, sought to escape responsibility for making the decision* and at the time told [Foreman] that he had heard the grievant arguing in a loud voice with another employee—as if to fortify [Foreman's] suspicions."

[3]"Substitution of Disciplinary Suspension for Discharge (A Proposed 'Guide to the Perplexed' in Arbitration)," *Arbitration Journal,* 35 (1980), pp. 27–28.

The result: When all the facts were in, it turned out that Workman had been upset with Foreman that morning because Foreman had passed him over unfairly (in his opinion) for a chance to train on a new and higher paying job. Not only did Workman's anger provide an explanation for the commotion he caused; his charge that Foreman had discriminated against him also gave Foreman a motive for accusing him of being drunk. Since the company had no other convincing evidence that Workman was under the influence, Workman's discharge was revoked.[4]

If Bolton, in this example, had stepped in as an in-house judge, or third party, and had heard both sides of the story, Workman might never have been discharged, and third-party intervention from the "outside"—in the person of the arbitrator—might not have been necessary.

[4]*Capital Area Transit Authority,* 69 LA 811, 813 (Ellman, 1977).

Chapter 5

PROOF

"At the investigation, did the 'judge' obtain substantial evidence or proof that the employee was guilty as charged?"

INTRODUCTION

Except for disputes involving chronic alcoholism, proof is probably the factor most frequently contested where discipline/discharge takes place for alcohol-related misconduct (i.e. intoxication, drinking, or possession of spirits on the job). The typical situation arises where the employer claims that the grievant was under the influence, or was drinking, or had some alcoholic beverage in his possession, and gets a flat denial in response.

As with all other discipline/discharge subjects, the employer must bear the *burden of proof* in a case of alcohol-related misconduct.

> *Arbitrator Witney:* "As countless arbitration decisions demonstrate, in a disciplinary case the employer bears the burden of proof. In short, the employer must supply convincing evidence that the employee committed the offense for which he was discharged. It is up to the employer to prove the employee 'guilty;' and not the employee who must prove himself 'not guilty.' "[1]

Quantum of Proof in Alcohol Cases

How much proof the employer must produce—or, as they say in the business, what *quantum of proof* is required in an alcohol case—

[1]*Midwest Telephone Co.,* 66 LA 311, 314 (Witney, 1976).

is less settled, and arbitrators do not present a united front on that question. There are three different standards for measuring the quantum of proof:

(1) the most stringent standard, *proof beyond a reasonable doubt;*

(2) the middle ground, *clear and convincing evidence;* and

(3) the least exacting standard, *preponderance of the evidence.*

In alcohol-related offenses (intoxication, drinking, or possession) where discharge is imposed, some arbitrators have held the company to the highest standard. Ordinarily they come to this approach through *one or both of two routes.*

First, those who adopt this standard generally rely in good part on the unfortunate effects that discharge will have on the employee. It is reasoned that discharge is the most drastic penalty an employee can suffer, depriving him of his livelihood, his seniority, and other vested interests in his job, and that an employee who has been fired for drinking or intoxication is likely to have a hard time finding another job, since a prospective employer may be reluctant to risk a repetition of such serious misconduct.[2] Moreover, "benefit of the doubt" and "presumption of innocence" are likely to play a greater part than in the case of the two other standards of proof.

As for the second route to "beyond a reasonable doubt," this standard, since it has much more of an absolutist cast than either of the two lesser standards, is most appealing to those who yearn for certainty and who are uneasy with sustaining a discharge unless the proof of guilt is water-tight.

[2]See, for example, Arbitrator Whyte: "In making this determination of fact—whether or not Grievant consumed intoxicants on the job—Company will be held to have had the burden of proving the allegation beyond a reasonable doubt. It is uniformly recognized that since discharge is the "capital punishment" of labor relations, and since employees discharged for serious offenses (and drinking on the job is a serious offense because it involves not only production but also safety of the accused employee and his co-workers) frequently find it impossible to find other employment, proof of his having committed the offense is subject to the most stringent standards." (*Greif Brothers Corp.*, 79–1 ARB ¶8244, 4014 (1979) (intoxication not proved).

Other cases in which the "beyond a reasonable doubt" standard is adopted include *Bi-State Development Agency,* 72 LA 198 (Newmark, 1979) (intoxication not proved; grievant reinstated, but without back pay in view of his refusal to take sobriety test); *Blaw-Knox Co.*, 66–2 ARB ¶8532 (S. Wood, 1966) (intoxication proved and discharge upheld); *Charleston Naval Shipyard,* 70–1 ARB ¶8301 (Kesselman, 1970) (intoxication proved though discharge found too severe because of grievant's long service and possibility his alcohol problem could be treated); *U.S. Pipe and Foundry Co.*, 77–2 ARB ¶8479 (J. King, 1977) (drinking not proved, discharge reduced to 90–day suspension since grievant was guilty only of bringing alcoholic beverage on company property); *Okonite Co.*, 74–2 ARB ¶8525 (Ludlum, 1974) (no proof grievants intended to bring beer into plant).

Many arbitrators disagree both with "the beyond a reasonable doubt" standard in alcohol-related misconduct cases and with the kind of thinking that is subsumed in the phrase "discharge is industrial capital punishment." Arbitrator R. Gibson points out that proof beyond a reasonable doubt properly applies mainly where the employee is charged with misconduct of a criminal nature (or misconduct involving moral turpitude). Intoxication may be a most serious matter in terms of maintaining order and safety at the workplace, but it certainly is not an offense of criminal character. Thus, the employer need only prove his case by a *preponderance of the evidence.*[3]

A number of arbitrators share that view.[4] Others require something more than a preponderance, but still less than proof beyond a reasonable doubt—i.e., *clear and convincing evidence.*[5]

Not only is there a lack of consensus among arbitrators concerning the three standards, but many are vague about exactly what standard they themselves have adopted in a particular case. An arbitrator may label the standard that he has adopted as "preponderance," for example, when he could have labeled it "clear and convincing" or even "beyond a reasonable doubt."[6] One reason why a certain amount of

[3]"Although proof beyond a reasonable doubt may be applicable to those cases involving moral turpitude such as theft, criminal rules of evidence do not automatically extend to the grievant in every disciplinary case, e.g., absenteeism, incompetence, negligence, intoxication and similar types of misconduct or deficiencies. Accordingly, the arbitrator finds that the Employer need only establish grounds for discipline by a preponderance of the credible evidence." (*Spartek, Inc.*, 77–1 ARB ¶8230, 4009 (1977))

[4]For other "preponderance" cases, see, e.g., *Cessna Aircraft Co.*, 52 LA 764 (Altrock, 1969) (discharge for drinking on job upheld); *Ward Furniture Manufacturing Co.*, 63–2 ARB ¶8826 (Boles, 1963) (employer proved grievant was drunk, but discharge overturned because of lax enforcement of rule against intoxication); *Alameda-Contra Costa Transit District*, 80–1 ARB ¶8060 (Randall, 1979) (intoxication proved, discharged sustained); *Black Diamond Enterprises, Inc.*, 52 LA 945, 69–2 ARB ¶8469 (Nicholas, 1969) (employer proved on-the-job drinking, discharge sustained); *Kast Metals Corp.*, 65 LA 783 (E. Davis, 1975) (no proof grievant was in possession of alcohol, reinstatement with back pay ordered).

[5]*Okonite Co.*, 74 LA 664 (Ghiz, 1980) (severity of discharge penalty cited as reason for adopting "clear and convincing" standard); *Kansas-Nebraska Natural Gas Co.*, 72–2 ARB ¶8493 (Helbing, 1972) (no proof of drunkenness, grievant reinstated with back pay); *McGraw-Edison Power System Div.*, 52 LA 825 (Volz, 1969) (proof of drinking but not intoxication, discharge reduced to suspension); *Reliance Electric Co.*, 76–2 ARB ¶8446 (Robert Gibson, 1976) (intoxication not proved, three-day suspension improper); *Park Haven Care Center*, 79–2 ARB ¶8328 (Fitzsimmons, 1979) (grievant not intoxicated but suffering adverse effects from medication, discharge reduced to suspension); *Diamond International Corp.*, 82–2 ARB ¶8326 (Ipavec, 1982) (possession of alcohol proved, suspension upheld).

[6]In *The Holliston Mills, Inc.*, 73–1 ARB ¶8177 (Simon, 1973), involving on-the-job intoxication, the arbitrator mentioned both the "clear and convincing" and "preponderance" tests; while in *W. R. Grace & Co.*, 69 LA 1071, 1074 (Flaten, 1977), "a great preponderance of the credible evidence," but not proof beyond a reasonable doubt, was required to sustain the grievant's discharge for drinking, because the situation had "some of the elements of a criminal case."

slipping and sliding from one quantum of proof to another goes on is that the three standards in the abstract do not lend themselves to precise definitions. Arbitrators draw conclusions about what is "clear and convincing" (or "preponderance" or "beyond a reasonable doubt") in reference to a particular set of facts. Facts that are "clear and convincing" to one arbitrator may be only a "preponderance" to another.

And so, since these standards are so imprecise, are they useful at all? A strong argument can be made that in their conventional form their usefulness is only marginal. If such standards are to be viable they cannot be thought of in quantitative terms or as precise "mathematical" measurements but instead must be viewed with "variable degrees of caution," as suggested by the West Coast panel of the National Academy of Arbitrators:

> "In that sense, then, an arbitrator may wish simply, on balance, to be more persuaded than not ('preponderance') in many cases; pretty certain in others ('clear and convincing'); and completely convinced in yet others ('beyond a reasonable doubt')."[7]

In some instances, arbitrators have met the problem of inexact definitions by throwing out the three-standard hierarchy altogether and requiring the company to prove its case by "substantial and competent" evidence or other basic criteria.[8]

Quantum of proof—a manager's perspective

From the manager's point of view, concrete disciplinary decisions have to be made when alcohol misconduct occurs, and his focus needs to be a pragmatic one. Ordinarily, he has little interest in fine and not immediately useful distinctions and would find it frustrating to try to figure out what some arbitrator down the line may say about a decision which may have been made under very demanding circumstances. Unlike the arbitrator, he also must take into account management's larger goals of maintaining authority and running the business effectively.

Thus, the technicalities of quantum of proof may not be as important to the manager and the supervisor as they are to the arbitrator

[7]"Problems of Proof: Report of the West Coast Area," in PROBLEMS OF PROOF IN ARBITRATION, Proceedings of the 19th Annual Meeting, National Academy of Arbitrators (Washington, D.C.: BNA Books, 1967), p. 195.

[8]*F. and M. Schaeffer Brewing Co.*, 68–2 ARB ¶8739, 5564 (Seidenberg, 1968), where a one-day suspension for reporting to work under the influence was upheld.

and the advocates in the arbitration business. Nonetheless, the manager, while primarily concerned with practical and immediate solutions to his problems, must also keep one eye on the arbitral function, with its unrelenting emphasis upon producing the proof. The manager functions at his peril if his actions are not free from the taint of arbitrariness; if his decisions are not backed by solid evidence; and if he makes a decision without taking all the available evidence into account. Within this equation, a feel for how much proof he will need becomes essential.

Direct and Circumstantial Evidence in Alcohol Cases

There are two types of evidence in cases of alcohol-related misconduct:

> *Direct evidence*—evidence that proves a fact directly; the "I saw him do it" type; and
>
> *Circumstantial evidence*—evidence of facts from which the fact to be proved can be inferred; the "He must have done it (even if I didn't see him do it) because x, y and z" type.

Both types of evidence are equally valuable and can be used successfully to prove the company's case provided that, in the case of *direct evidence,* the evidence is *credible,* or believable; and, in the case of *circumstantial evidence,* that the inference *follows logically from the facts* and *the facts themselves are solidly established.*

The three basic types of alcohol-related misconduct differ somewhat as to the type of evidence normally used as proof.

Intoxication is almost always established by direct evidence, such as a report by one or more supervisors that he (they) saw an employee showing signs of being under the influence—the smell of alcohol on his breath, glassy eyes, unsteady gait, and so on.

Drinking and possession of alcoholic beverages are proved by either direct *or* circumstantial evidence. Someone may spot an employee taking a drink or carrying a can of beer into the plant. But even without an eye-witness account, drinking can still be proved if, e.g., a supervisor walks into a locker room and sees the employee tossing an empty beer can into a trash can; the can is still cold and dripping moisture; and the employee has the smell of alcohol on his breath. Possession can be established if, for example, booze is found in an employee's locker to which no one else has a key.

The remainder of this chapter is concerned with what adds up to proof—and what does not—with respect to each of the three types of alcohol misconduct—intoxication, drinking, and possession.

I. INTOXICATION

> "The man had been boozing"—"He was drunk as a skunk"—"He was in his cups"—"You could tell he'd had a belt or two"—"He was soused"—"He must have killed a pint easy"—"Maybe he wasn't falling down, but he sure was a little tight"

WHAT DOES BEING "INTOXICATED" MEAN?

Or, to put it another way, what exactly does the employer have to prove?

In everyday parlance, nice distinctions are made among the degrees to which an individual's mind and body become affected by alcohol. To say that someone is "tight" or "tipsy," for example, usually implies that he shows some signs of having been drinking but has not lost control of his physical or mental faculties to a significant degree. To say that someone is "drunk," "intoxicated," or "inebriated," on the other hand, indicates that he has lost physical coordination and mental coherence. The even stronger slang terms "blotto," "soused," and "stewed" describe an individual whose condition is just short of passing out.

But at the workplace, distinctions made in everyday life do not play an important part. Distinctions *are* made among the three types of alcohol-related offenses: intoxication, drinking, and possession of alcoholic beverages. But "degrees" of intoxication are not generally recognized.

If an employee is affected by alcohol to an appreciable degree, he is said to be "intoxicated" or "under the influence"—the catch-all phrases. He need not be "falling down drunk" or stumbling over his machine before the employer may take disciplinary action.[9] The em-

[9]"It is certainly not necessary to be falling down drunk to be intoxicated. The slightest degree of intoxication creates an extreme hazard to the employee involved, his fellow employees and the property of the Company." (*Magma Copper Co.*, 64–2 ARB ¶8439, 4569 (T. Roberts, 1964)) In *Northrop Worldwide Services, Inc.*, 64 LA 743, 748–9 (Goodstein, 1975), the arbitrator cited with approval the opinion of Arbitrator Geissinger in *Page Aircraft Maintenance, Inc.*, 56 LA 860 (1971), ". . . that the Rule permits of no other construction than that a finding of 'under the influence'—no matter how heavily or lightly under the rule—requires mandatory discharge." See also *Golden Foundry, Inc.*, 76–1 ARB ¶8012 (Traynor, 1975).

ployer is entitled to discipline employees for intoxication not only to penalize poor work performance but also to prevent such problems from occurring.[10]

In recognition of the fact that even an employee who is just slightly "high" or "happy" or "tight" can be a potential problem, some contracts or company rules—particularly in industries like transportation, where sobriety is critical—put employees on explicit notice that being under "the slightest influence of alcohol" will lead to discipline;[11] or that employees must be "free from any effect produced by alcoholic beverages";[12] or that "no degree of intoxication will be tolerated."[13]

Still, at least some degree of intoxication must be proved. Not every employee who has a couple of beers before work and shows up with alcohol on his breath is going to be appreciably affected by those beers.

> *Arbitrator Carnes:* "The rule requires that an employee be *under* the influence of alcohol—that is, the influence must be more than a merely detectable one, it must be *an appreciable influence which adversely affects the capacity of the employee to competently perform his or her job duties in a safe manner*" (emphasis added).[14]

For purposes of judging when an employee has crossed over that sometimes fine line from sobriety to intoxication, arbitrators have recognized the validity of two kinds of evidence: *direct evidence*—what supervisors see and hear; and *physical evidence*—measurements of blood alcohol levels.

[10]The same logic is used to support the employer's right to discipline employees for drinking on the job.

[11]*Alameda-Contra Costa Transit District,* 80–1 ARB ¶8060 (Randall, 1979).

[12]*Hughes Air Corp.,* 76–1 ARB ¶8169 (Wyckoff, 1976).

[13]*McGraw-Edison Power Systems, Div.,* 52 LA 825 (Volz, 1969).

[14]*General Felt Industries, Inc.,* 74 LA 972, 976 (Carnes, 1979). Arbitrator Volz: "An employee may be said to be under the influence of alcohol when, through the intentional use of alcohol, he lessens his ability to perform satisfactorily his duties throughout the workday, including a reasonable period of overtime, with safety to himself, to his fellow employees, and the equipment and product." (*Altamil Corp.,* 71–1 ARB ¶8199 (1971)) Arbitrator Sass: "In the opinion of the Arbitrator, the terms 'unfit condition' and 'intoxicated condition' imply something more than just the fact that an individual has had a few drinks. They imply that the individual has had enough to drink close enough to work time to adversely affect his judgment and job performance." (*Consolidation Coal Co.,* 82–2 ARB ¶8605, 5705 (1982)). See also *Capital Area Transit Authority,* 69 LA 811 (Ellman, 1977); *Koppers Co.,* 65–1 ARB ¶8013 (Loucks, 1964) (being "hung over" and being under the influence not the same).

DIRECT EVIDENCE

> "I am slow of speech and of a slow tongue." (Exodus IV:10)

Intoxication is one of the few areas where nonexpert, lay opinion is admissible as evidence, not only in arbitration proceedings but in courts of law in many states as well. In some instances the union may protest that discipline cannot reasonably be based on anything as "subjective" as a supervisor's judgment, without the "objective" corroboration of a blood alcohol test.[15] But that argument will rarely prevail (see below, p. 74). It may be true, as one arbitrator has commented, that "the determination of whether or not an employee was 'under the influence' of alcohol is never an easy task."[16] Nevertheless, a supervisor's judgment as to whether an employee is under the influence will normally be admitted and, as a rule, given considerable weight by an arbitrator *if* formed on the basis of specific, complete, and credible observation of the employee's behavior and appearance. In fact, in most cases involving discipline for intoxication that come before arbitrators, the "proof" presented by the company consists of *observations* of what supervisors saw the grievant do or heard him say, on the basis of which the supervisor formed an *opinion* that the grievant was under the influence.

Arbitrator Ross: "It does not take an expert to render a relevant and acceptable opinion on intoxication."[17]

Arbitrator Rose: "Drinking men are generally fair judges of intoxication."[18]

[15]See Note 18 for case citations.

[16]*General Felt Industries, Inc.*, Note 14 above.

[17]*Cal Custom/Hawk*, 65 LA 723 (1975).

[18]*Freightliner Corporation*, KEY CASES IN DETAIL. Cases in agreement include *F. and M. Schaeffer Brewing Co.*, 68–2 ARB ¶8739 (Seidenberg, 1968); *Blaw-Knox Co.*, 66–2 ARB ¶8532 (S. Wood, 1966); *Hi-Life Packing Co.*, 41 LA 1083 (Sembower, 1983); *Tennessee River Pulp & Paper Co.*, 68 LA 421 (Simon, 1976); *City of Buffalo, 59 LA 334 (Rinaldo, 1972); Sherwin-Williams Co.*, 66 LA 273 (Rezler, 1976). In *Active Products Co.*, 68–1 ARB ¶8103, 3371 (May, 1967), the arbitrator noted that union arguments about the incompetence of supervisors to judge whether an employee is intoxicated suffered from a fatal inconsistency: "The Union members chose to make judgments that the Grievant was not drunk, albeit he admitted that he had been drinking while the Company men maintained that he was under the influence of alcohol. If the Company maintains no experts in the field of intoxication, it might reasonably be concluded that neither does the Union and therefore the judgment is equally bad on the part of one as one the part of the other. It is, however, my conviction that a reasonable man under reasonable circumstances can judge the condition of a person as being intoxicated or not being intoxicated by his actions, his talk, etc."

DIRECT EVIDENCE: A PREVIEW

What the supervisor needs to know:

- *Accepted symptoms of intoxication*—what makes a credible case?
- *Typical problems with supervisors' reports*—where direct evidence can fall down
  1. The "single symptom" problem
  2. Key symptom missing
  3. Delayed reactions
  4. The "opportunity factor"
  5. Conflicting, inconsistent, vague, and otherwise incredible testimony
- *Three classic defenses against intoxication charges*
  1. "It's my medication!"
  2. "I'm sick!"
  3. "It's those fumes!"

Accepted Symptoms of Intoxication

> *Arbitrator Cantor:* "The common denominators of intoxication are thickness of speech, lack of coordination and body movement and the presence of alcohol about the person."[19]

Credibility is the key to direct evidence. Direct evidence can serve as persuasive proof of intoxication only if it is credible—i.e., if it can be believed. The credibility of a supervisor's judgment that an employee was under the influence hinges on whether his observations of

[19] *Modern Bakery, Inc.,* 70–2 ARB ¶8599 (1970) See also *Hunt Foods and Industries, Inc.,* 64–3 ARB ¶8960, 6318 (Hebert, 1964); "The employee's conduct, his demeanor, his appearance, evidence of a flushed face, a glassy eye, an unsteady gait, slowness of movement, the smell of intoxicating liquor on the breath are all circumstances to be considered in passing on the question of whether an employee is drunk or under the influence of intoxication." *General Felt Industries, Inc.,* Note 14 above: "Classical signs of intoxication" include "speech—thick, slurred, loud; flushed face; general appearance—dishevelment, dirtiness, unkemptness; appearance of eyes—red, watery, heavy lids; fixed pupils; breath—foul, distinctive odor of various intoxicants; gait—walking unsteadily, deliberately and overcarefully, swaying, weaving, stooped; behavior—excessive silliness or boisterousness, etc."

the employee's behavior and appearance correspond to the accepted symptoms of intoxication listed below:

> *Odor*—The smell of alcohol is evident on the individual's breath or around his person.
>
> *Speech*—The individual's speech may be described as "thick"; abnormally slow; slurred; incoherent; disfigured in any way.
>
> *Appearance*—Glassy or bloodshot eyes; flushed or red-faced.
>
> *Movement*—Uncoordinated; clumsy. The individual weaves or staggers; moves in a very slow or deliberate manner; is wobbly and unsteady on his feet.
>
> *Manner*—Boisterous, loud, profane, belligerent; or unusually quiet, lethargic—in any event, different from the individual's normal manner.

As a general rule, the more of these symptoms an employee exhibits, and the more pronounced those symptoms appear to be, the more credible a supervisor's judgment that the employee was under the influence will be.[20] In one case, the grievant was done in by supervisors' observations that he was "very unsteady . . . swaying around"; that liquor was detected on his breath; that his "face seemed flushed, eyes glassy . . . tongue couldn't seem to speak the word plain."[21] In another, the decisive evidence was that he had "constricted pupils and a disheveled appearance, his shirt was out, his speech was slurred, his breath had an odor of alcohol, and he was so drowsy that he would fall asleep in his chair."[22]

[20]Arbitrator Carnes: "Judgment is exercised in response to the totality of the observed circumstances. The greater the number and more pronounced the signs, the greater the assumption of greater alcoholic influence and performance impairment." (*General Felt Industries, Inc.*, Note 14 above) In *Magnavox, Co.*, 29 LA 305, 310 (H. Dworkin, 1957), the arbitrator listed the accepted signs of intoxication, then noted, "While none of these are conclusive in any particular case, it might be said generally that being under the influence of liquor contemplates proof of loss of control of one's physical and mental faculties to some appreciable degree."

[21]*Ward Furniture Manufacturing Co.*, 63–2 ARB ¶8826, 5661 (Boles, 1963).

[22]*Charleston Naval Shipyard*, 70–1 ARB ¶8301, 3996 (Kesselman, 1970). See also (among many other cases where intoxication has been proved by direct evidence) *Chrysler Corp.*, 40 LA 935 (Alexander, 1963) (grievant was "staggering or weaving . . . glassy-eyed . . . breath smelled of alcohol . . . speech was not clear"); *Parkview-Gem, Inc.*, 59 LA 429, 431 (Dugan, 1972) (grievant had "alcoholic odor about him," spoke with a slurred and loud voice, abusive tone); *Cities Service Co.*, 77 LA 1180, 1184 (Brisco, 1982) (grievant showed "evidence of loud talking, resting her head on her forearms, shielding her mouth with her hands, not replying audibly as was her habit, walking slowly while holding the stair rail with both hands, failure to commence work, and the smell of alcohol on her breath"); *Alameda-Contra Costa Transit District*, 80–1 ARB ¶8060, 3274 (Randall, 1979) ("strong smell of alcohol . . . eyes were red . . . speech weak and 'fuzzy' . . . skin pale and dry looking . . . unreasonable").

A supervisor's opinion carries especially great weight where he is familiar with the employee's normal behavior and on that basis can state competently that the employee was not his usual self. Thus, in one case, the arbitrator brushed aside union protests that loud and boisterous language do not necessarily prove intoxication by pointing out that the two supervisors who concluded that the grievant was under the influence were familiar with his general demeanor and work habits and would not likely have been mistaken.[23]

Typical Problems With Supervisors' Reports

Where direct evidence falls short of proving that an employee was under the influence, the reason typically is not that the employer's witnesses did not "see what they saw." It's that what they saw did not add up to intoxication, in the arbitrator's judgment.

Here are six major problems that come up in direct evidence cases:

1. *The "single symptom" problem*

The presence of one of the usual symptoms of intoxication, standing alone, may be misleading and should be investigated carefully. The *odor of alcohol* is the most troublesome. In combination with other symptoms (thickness of speech, an unmistakable stagger, etc.), alcohol on the breath is usually a reliable sign of intoxication.

Caveat: But when the solitary symptom is the smell of alcohol, then the employee's plea ("It's only cough syrup!" or "I just had a swallow—I'm not drunk!") may be valid.[24] The smell of alcohol somewhere on the employee's person and not specifically on his breath needs to be

[23]*F. and M. Schaeffer Brewing Co.*, 68–2 ARB ¶8739 (Seidenberg, 1968). See also *Tennessee River Pulp & Paper Co.*, 68 LA 421, 430 (Simon, 1976): "It has been held by more than one arbitrator that supervisors who have no medical training are capable of recognizing when an employee is intoxicated or under the influence of an alcoholic beverage if they objectively compare an employee's normal demeanor and work habits with those at the time that his sobriety is questioned." (Same principle cited in *Sherwin-Williams Co.*, 66 LA 273 (Rezler, 1976). In *Consolidation Coal Co.*, 82–2 ARB ¶8605 (Sass, 1982), the arbitrator discounted union testimony that a red complexion, glassy eyes, and difficult speech were usual for the grievant on the ground that his supervisors also were well acquainted with the grievant and knew what he normally looked like, yet did not normally suspect him of being under the influence.

[24]As in *McGraw-Edison Power Systems Div.*, 52 LA 825, (Volz, 1969), where the arbitrator stated, "where the only evidence consists of testimony of odor on the breath and a conclusion that it smelled like alcohol, but the employee acts and performs normally . . . no penalty is generally indicated" Similarly, Arbitrator H. Dworkin: "It is the judgment of the arbitrator that the presence of an odor of alcohol on one's breath would not in and of itself warrant a penalty of discharge since such condition is not synonymous with being under the influence . . . nor does it denote any impairment of one's physical and mental faculties." (*Magnavox Co.*, 29 LA 305, 310 (1957).

treated with special caution, especially in plants where industrial alcohol or similar-smelling products are used in production or even in cleaning.[25]

EXAMPLE: *"I could smell the booze—I knew he was drunk."*

Harry Workman is discharged for reporting to work with alcohol on his breath, even though his behavior is not erratic in any way. Miles Foreman's position: "As far as I am concerned, if a person has the smell on his breath, then he's under the influence."

The outcome: The arbitrator found that Miles Foreman had jumped to conclusions. Harry Workman had been drinking the night before, and, although the smell lingered on, tests showed that the level of alcohol in his blood was much lower than any reasonable standard would define as being under the influence.[26]

Alcohol on the breath may occur most frequently, but other single symptoms—boisterousness,[27] lack of coordination,[28] and a disheveled appearance[29]—have also been mistakenly equated with intoxication when they really were inspired by other causes.

SUPPOSE: *Mr. Excitable*

Harry Workman is discharged for being intoxicated after he is accused by one of his employer's customers of ramming a truck into a loading dock and breaking a loading plate. Harry became so excitable after the dock incident and spoke so incoherently that the customer concluded he must be drunk and called the company.

The outcome: All witnesses (including General Manager Powers) testified that at *all* times when Workman became excited, he spoke rapidly and disjointedly so that he could barely be understood. Even at the hearing his speech was so indistinct and slurred that the Arbitrator could hardly understand the testimony! Since Powers had also agreed that

[25]See the arbitrator's reasoning in *Kansas-Nebraska Gas Co.,* KEY CASES IN DETAIL.

[26]*Memphis Light, Gas & Water Division,* 66 LA 948 (Rayson, 1976).

[27]*General Felt Industries, Inc.,* Note 14 above.

[28]*Reliance Electric Co.,* 76–2 ARB ¶8446 (Gibson, 1976), where the grievant's shaking, shivering, and poor coordination could have been explained by exposure to cold and an unexpected rainstorm on the way to work.

[29]*Western Air Lines, Inc.,* 37 LA 130 (Wyckoff, 1961), where flight attendant's disheveled appearance could have been due to the fact that she overslept and dressed for work hurriedly, rather than to preflight drinking.

Workman's gait was steady, his face was not flushed, and there was no smell of alcohol on his breath, the arbitrator refused to uphold the discharge.[30]

An individual who behaves excitedly or who has alcohol on his breath may fit a particular supervisor's conception of how a drunken person is supposed to look or act. But if the supervisor takes action on the basis of his personal attitudes, without making an adequate investigation and without taking into account the objective standards described in the preceding section, his judgment will be vulnerable to charges by the union that it was "purely subjective" and should be set aside.

2. *Key symptom missing*

On the other side of the coin, the absence of alcohol on the breath, or of some other major symptom, may also lead an arbitrator to doubt that an employee was really under the influence. Absence of a major symptom (such as difficulty in walking) tends to loom especially large if the employee is described as having been in an advanced state of drunkenness in which that symptom would normally be expected.[31] But a supervisor's failure to report a particular symptom can hurt the company in another way as well.

SUPPOSE: *"I didn't know he had a wooden leg."*

The night superintendent, Lem Bolton, asserts that Harry Workman appeared glassy-eyed and had beer on his breath. Yet he is unable to say whether Workman wobbled or staggered—despite the fact that he had ample opportunity to observe Workman's behavior.

The arbitrator's reaction: It is "difficult to understand how a member of management could walk 50 to 60 feet from the work area to his office, talk to the Grievant for about 15 or 20 minutes . . . walk with him from the office to an automobile, walk from an automobile to the emergency room of the hospital and back to the automobile; upon return to the plant walk back to the office *and never observe* his walk, never saw him stagger or weave; in fact he could not even testify how the employee walked."[32]

[30]*Blue Diamond Co.*, 66 LA 1136 (Summers, 1976). Another case in which the grievant's "normal" behavior was not taken into account is *Greif Brothers Corp., Seymour & Peck Division, Charlotte, N.C.*, 79–1 ARB ¶8244 (Whyte, 1979), where the grievant often used profane language and worked at a slow pace; see KEY CASES IN DETAIL.

[31]The fact that no one observed the grievant walking unsteadily or showing other signs of poor physical coordination also contributed to the arbitrator's conclusion that intoxication was not proved in *Greif Brothers Corp.*, Note 30 above.

[32]*The Holliston Mills, Inc.*, 73–1 ARB ¶8177, 3659–60 (Simon, 1973).

This case illustrates how, in some cases, a missing symptom in a supervisor's report can lead an arbitrator to conclude that a supervisor *just wasn't very observant* and, on that basis, to question the reliability of his testimony as a whole.

3. *Delayed reaction*

Almost nothing hurts a supervisor's credibility more than a delay in taking action on a suspected case of intoxication. It must be presumed that if a supervisor lets an employee go to work, or continue working, he has concluded that the employee is sober and can do his job.

EXAMPLE: *"Actions speak louder than words"*

> During her shift Helen Workman, a cocktail waitress, gets into a series of hassles with Miles Foreman over a disputed work assignment, and Foreman has to tell her repeatedly to get back to work and do her job. Finally, Foreman has had enough. He concludes on the basis of Workman's loud and angry manner, as well as a smell of alcohol on her breath, that she is drunk and sends her home. Workman is discharged as a result.
>
> *The problem with Foreman's testimony:* "If [Workman] was clearly and obviously intoxicated and could not perform her job, it was most unlikely that [Foreman] would have ordered her over and over to return to work. Indeed, by doing so, it is apparent that he did not consider her condition to be as serious as the Company now says it is. It is even possible that by ordering her to return to work, [Foreman] let us say essentially 'waived' drinking as a basis for discharge at that point."[33]

4. *The "opportunity factor"*

When a supervisor detects signs of intoxication during working hours, especially if the symptoms are not particularly blatant, he must recognize that the employee could only have done his drinking either *off premises,* before work or during a break; or *on premises* in the course

[33]*Sahara Hotel,* 76–2 ARB ¶8410 (Koven, 1976). In *Continental Can Co.,* 76–1 ARB ¶8006, 4532 (Sembower, 1975), several supervisors not only permitted but urged the grievant to continue working on a technically difficult operation, even after one of them had been warned that he appeared to be drunk. "If indeed the Grievant was as intoxicated as some of the Company's testimony would indicate, this indeed is amazing supervisory conduct." See also *Super Valu Stores, Inc.,* 60 LA 652, 654 (Doyle, 1973) (supervisor to whom grievant reported at beginning of shift testified he could smell beer or alcohol on grievant's breath but added, "He didn't act unusual to me." *Standard Beverage, Inc.,* 52 LA 989 (Koven, 1969) (grievant sounded "strange" but plant manager did not think that he was intoxicated and authorized him to work extra half hour of overtime)

of his shift. If it can be shown that it just was not possible for the employee to have been drinking either off premises or on premises, despite whatever symptoms to the contrary he seemed to present, then discipline for intoxication will normally not stand up.

On premises: The major question about intoxication due to drinking on premises is *opportunity*. Employees do not ordinarily drink openly, where it would be easy to get caught. Thus, a supervisor who accuses an employee of being under the influence has to be prepared to meet the protest, "No way! I never had a chance to drink!"

***EXAMPLE:** Where or when?*

Harry Workman is discharged for being under the influence when Miles Foreman observes him moving very slowly and speaking with a slur around 4:00 p.m. Harry admits bringing a can of beer into the plant but denies that he had even a sip.

The outcome: Negative for the company. When Workman clocked in at 1:30 p.m., no one noticed anything wrong with his behavior. From that point until 4:00, no evidence was produced that he ever left his job operating a crane, and thus, he would not have had the opportunity to do any drinking.[34]

ASK YOURSELF:

At the location or locations where he was working, is it likely that other people would have seen him if he had been drinking, or could he have taken a surreptitious "belt"? *or*

Was the employee missing from his workplace long enough to go to the locker room, restroom, or other area where he could have some privacy to drink? *or*

Was a bottle or other physical evidence of drinking found where the employee had access to it?[35]

[34] *U.S. Pipe & Foundry Co.*, 77–2 ARB ¶8479 (King, 1977).

[35] As in *Ward Funiture Mfg. Co.*, 63–2 ARB ¶8826 (Boles, 1963), where four empty and one half-empty vodka bottles were found in an out-of-the-way area that the grievant had been seen entering on the day he was accused of being intoxicated. Or *Dayton-Walther Co.*, 77 LA 1064, 1067 (Traynor, 1981): "Coupled with the grievant's actions leading to the belief that he was intoxicated and his going to a locker which was not assigned to him, and which in fact did contain vodka, is just one more indication that if he hadn't had anything to drink before coming to work, there was ample opportunity for him between 5:30 A.M. and 6:00 A.M. to have gone to the locker room and imbibed."

Off premises: If an employee has not had a chance to drink at work, then logically he must have become intoxicated before reporting—either before his shift or during a break. Where off-premises drinking is the issue, *the following problems* may arise: A supervisor has spoken with or observed the employee at the time he reports in, or shortly thereafter, and notices nothing wrong; or a supervisor does indeed detect some sign that the employee may be under the influence but nonetheless lets him go to work or to continue working.

Either way, the employee can make a good case that he could not have been intoxicated when he reported, and the company will find itself up against the "opportunity factor" with nowhere to go.

SUPPOSE: *A whiskey breath—but not too bad*

> About an hour and a half into his shift, a supervisor smells alcohol on Harry Workman's breath, finds him behaving erratically, and concludes that he is intoxicated.
>
> *The problem:* Where or when? *On premises?* No one saw Workman take a drink or leave the composing room between the time he clocked in and the time he was sent home. *Off premises?* When he clocked in, Workman was observed by Miles Foreman to be "extra jovial," although not flushed; Lem Bolton noticed whiskey on his breath, but thought he seemed "OK."
>
> *The outcome:* Almost inevitable. "It seems reasonable to conclude that if [the supervisor] smelled whiskey on [Workman's] breath and let him go to work then [the supervisor] must have felt that [he] was not under the influence of intoxicating liquor."[36]

5. *Conflicting, inconsistent, vague, and otherwise incredible testimony*

> *Arbitrator Allman:* "The charge of drunkenness is a serious one. . . . It is well established that mere opinion evidence is not sufficient. The evidence must be sufficiently specific in describing various details of appearance and conduct so that it is clear that the person accused is under the influence of liquor."[37]

A clear case that an employee was under the influence has at least several essential features: The case is based on facts, i.e., witnesses' specific and credible observations; it is internally consistent; and it leaves no major questions unanswered. In short, it "hangs together," "makes sense."

[36] *Washington, D.C., Publishers Association,* 70–2 ARB ¶8463 (Buckwalter, 1970).
[37] *Genest-Midwest, Inc.,* 67–2 ARB ¶8569, 4993 (1967).

By contrast, where company witnesses cannot agree on how the employee looked or behaved, or even on whether he was intoxicated at all;[38] where a material witness is not called;[39] or where a witness testifies about feelings rather than facts, the arbitrator is likely to be left with a confused picture of what really took place. *The Holliston Mills* case offers a prime example of a case that is built on this kind of shifting ground.[40]

- Whereas one supervisor, who saw the grievant for just a few moments, testified that "he was unstable in his walking, too, some, when he walked," the night superintendent, who was with the grievant for several hours, noticed nothing wrong with his walk.
- Moreover, the night superintendent's behavior was indecisive and self-contradictory. At the time of the incident, he reportedly told the foreman, "I *think* I have a guy here who has been drinking and I *feel* like I should take him to the hospital." But the reprimand notice he later wrote up stated, "I was *at once aware* that you were under the influence of an intoxicant," and "your actions and appearance *left no doubt* that you were under the influence." (emphasis added).
- Finally, the night superintendent testified that he smelled beer on the grievant's breath from a distance of several feet; yet he failed to notice the much stronger odor of thinner and color mix in the area, which other witnesses—both company and union—said pervaded the plant at the time.

  Outcome: This kind of testimony "failed miserably" to convince the arbitrator that the grievant was intoxicated.

[38]As in *Capital Area Transit Authority,* 69 LA 811, 814 (Ellman, 1977), where the grievant was discharged after his foreman concluded he was under the influence; at the hearing, however, the foreman's supervisor, who had also observed the grievant, admitted that he had detected nothing wrong with his behavior, and a third supervisor who might have backed up the foreman's judgment was not called to testify. Foreman's own statements were also inconsistent in that he testified that Workman was moving with "a little off-balance sway"—"hardly the kind of drunken stagger which he and the employer thereafter sought to paint it," as the arbitrator noted. See also *Trans World Airlines,* 38 LA 1221 (Wallen, 1962).

[39]Two witnesses called by the company testified that the grievant had alcohol on his breath, but neither observed any other manifestation of impaired ability, and "[s]everal witnesses who might have shed some further light on grievant's condition were not called to testify at the hearing." The arbitrator found that intoxication was not proved. (*Bi-State Development Agency,* 72 LA 198, 204 (Newmark, 1979))

[40]Cited Note 32 above.

6. *The hearsay problem*

> Hearsay is testimony given (or a statement made) by a person who reports not what he knows, but what he has heard from someone else, for the purpose of proving the truth of the matter stated.

TAKE A HYPOTHETICAL:

Dick Sargent, a plant gate guard, turns Harry Workman away one morning after concluding that he's drunk. He phones Personnel Director Dave Powers to tell him what he has observed and follows up with a written report: "Workman reeked of whiskey, could hardly stand up, and put up an argument when told to leave the premises." At the arbitration hearing, Powers testifies about what Sargent told him and offers his written report as evidence—but Sargent himself is no longer with the company, and is not present to testify about what he saw.

Powers' testimony is a classic example of *hearsay*.[41] In a court of law, hearsay (with certain recognized exceptions) is customarily excluded from evidence. The reason: Its validity depends not only upon the credibility of the person testifying about what he was told, but upon the credibility of his informant—whose accuracy and truthfulness cannot be tested by cross-examination, that "great engine of truth."[42]

The regular rules of evidence are not "necessarily" observed in arbitration, and most arbitrators will admit hearsay evidence into the record. But because of its inherent weaknesses, it will not normally be given much weight, and whenever the crucial part of the company's case rests on hearsay, discipline cannot be expected to stand up.[43]

[41]For a full treatment of hearsay, see chapter on "Hearsay" in PROOF.

[42]*Phillips Painting Contractors,* 72 LA 16 (Brisco, 1978).

[43]See *Kansas-Nebraska Natural Gas Co.,* KEY CASES IN DETAIL, where the employee who originally reported seeing the grievant come in to work under the influence was not called to testify, even though "he was in the best position to evaluate the grievant's appearance and conduct. . . . Because the Company has the burden of proof it was incumbent upon it to produce [D] as a witness." In *Koppers Co.,* 65–1 ARB ¶8013 (Loucks, 1964), the arbitrator was unimpressed by a supervisor's testimony that a physician who examined the grievant concluded he was under the influence, where the physician himself did not testify and the company gave no reason for not producing him. In *Park Haven Care Center, Inc.,* 79–2 ARB ¶8328, 4375 (Fitzsimmons, 1979), the arbitrator gave little weight to unverified statements of certain witnesses "in view of the fact that the Company could have brought these witnesses to the hearing or made provisions to have their depositions taken . . . but the Company did not see fit to do so."

Three Classic Defenses Against Intoxication Charges

"It's my medication!"—"I'm sick!"—
"It's those fumes!"

A common pattern

The same pattern emerges in each of these three defenses: An employee is confronted with the charge that he's under the influence; he does not deny that he shows the *symptoms* of being intoxicated; instead, he claims that the *cause* of the symptoms was not excessive drinking but medication, illness, or some sort of industrial product—for none of which is he to blame or can he be blamed.

In some instances, the employee may be right. Common experience demonstrates that the smell of alcohol on the breath, uncoordinated movement, and slurred or "thick" speech represent the "common denominators" of intoxication; but common experience may be wrong. Many of the usual symptoms of drunkenness *may* also be produced by certain kinds of medication or illness; by fumes from industrial products; even by anger or other emotional upset.

Thorough investigation is critical in such cases. When an employee is suspected of being under the influence and claims his symptoms had some cause other than alcohol, the supervisor needs to take a hard look at the employee's defense—as the arbitrator certainly will.

There is a saying in the medical profession: "Common things happen most commonly." And so it is that more often than not, the symptoms of intoxication are generated by alcoholic beverages. If another explanation is put forward, it is up to the employee to produce *convincing evidence* to back up his explanation. Merely to raise the possibility that a particular drug or disease *could* have produced the symptoms in question is not enough; the evidence must definitely show that the disease or drug in fact produced those symptoms on the occasion in question.

The "medication defense"

When an employee protests that he was "under the influence" of medication, not alcohol—

ASK YOURSELF:

(The more "yes" answers, the more evidence that the employee's "defense" is valid.)

- Can the employee produce either the medication in question or a doctor's confirmation that he was taking medication?
- Does medical opinion confirm the employee's claim that the medication is likely to produce whatever symptoms of "intoxication" have been observed?[44]
- Has the employee suffered from the same or similar side effects on other occasions?
- Has the employee really been ill or injured?
- Has the employee previously told any management representative that he is taking a drug that might produce adverse side effects?

The following examples suggest how an arbitrator might deal with a "medication defense" type of case.

EXAMPLE NO. 1: Pills on the Q.T.

No one challenged Harry Workman's testimony that he was taking a prescription drug for treatment of tuberculosis when he was discharged for on-the-job intoxication, or that he had taken more than his usual dose on the day in question.

1. Workman asked permission to go home earlier in the day because he was feeling dizzy and unwell.

2. Miles Foreman let Workman stay on the job even after he reported that he was not feeling well.

3. Workman had not told management in advance that he might experience some problems from his medication.

The result: Workman's claim was accepted by the arbitrator. But the arbitrator decided that Workman was partly at fault for the misunderstanding as to whether or not he was intoxicated, and withheld back pay for that reason.[45]

[44]Denenberg and Denenberg, in ALCOHOL AND DRUGS: ISSUES IN THE WORKPLACE (Washington, D.C.: BNA Books, 1983), describe the symptoms of a number of common "tranquilizers," painkillers, and other psychogenic drugs that may be prescribed by doctors at p. 147.

[45]*Continental Can Co.*, 76–1 ARB ¶8006 (Sembower, 1975).

EXAMPLE NO. 2: Donnatal or several cans of beer

Harry Workman, a truck driver, was discharged for driving under the influence. He claimed his symptoms of intoxication were actually produced by Donnatal, a prescription drug. However:

1. The company physician stated in writing that Donnatal would not lead to drowsiness if taken in prescribed doses.

2. Though Workman's own doctor confirmed that Workman was taking the drug, he did not mention drowsiness as one of its side effects.

3. Workman did not pull off the highway when he stated he first felt the effects of the drug.

4. He acknowledged he had never been adversely affected by the medication either before or after the incident for which he was fired.

5. He did not mention his medication or illness to the highway patrolman who stopped him after his truck ran off the road, and who reached the conclusion that he had been drinking.

6. Workman also failed to account satisfactorily for several cans of beer found at the scene of his accident.

The result: Medication defense rejected.[46]

EXAMPLE NO. 3: A heady mixture

1. Although company witnesses reported smelling alcohol around Workman's person, the nurse and doctor who examined him later at the hospital smelled nothing.

2. Workman unquestionably was suffering from a bad cold or flu and had asked not to work that day.

[46]*Midwest Machinery Movers, Inc.*, 69–2 ARB ¶8564 (Kennedy, 1969). See also *Freightliner Corp.*, KEY CASES IN DETAIL, where the grievant did not deny that he had been drinking when he was informed "you don't belong here in this condition" and did not explain why his medication would have caused unsteady behavior on the date he was accused of drunkenness but not previously.

Other cases where the "medication defense" was rejected include: *Maule Industries, Inc.*, 66–2 ARB ¶8507 (Black, 1966) (company's expert medical witness established that amount of cough syrup and paragoric grievant claimed he had taken could not begin to account for blood alcohol level of 0.075 percent); *Schaefer-Alabama Corp.*, 70 LA 956 (LaValley, 1978) (grievant's own physician stated that dose of Darvon was "a little stronger than two aspirins"—not enough to cause vomiting and passing out); *FMC Corp.*, 83–1 ARB ¶8324 (Reynolds, 1983) (testimony of registered nurse that grievant was under influence of alcohol and drugs more credible than grievant's claim that symptoms were caused by combination of two beers the night before work and one 5 mg. valium pill the morning he was taken off job); *Capital Area Transit Authority*, 69 LA 811 (Ellman, 1977) (grievant's claim that he was suffering from strep throat and was taking Pertussin, a cough syrup containing alcohol, not credible since it was first made at arbitration hearing); *Somerset Bus Co., Inc.*, 73–1 ARB ¶8110 (Kerrison, 1973) (grievant's claim that symptoms were due to combination of fatigue, blood pressure medication, and sudden appearance of "unknown hijacker" completely unbelievable); *Mohawk Rubber Co.*, 47 LA 1029 (Teple, 1966) (aspirin compound not strong enough to explain grievant's falling asleep on job).

3. He was taking both over-the-counter and prescription drugs for his ailment. Workman's symptoms of "intoxication" showed up at the end of a week in which he worked 60 hours—10–11 of them that day.

4. Since Workman had an overall flawless work record and no history of on-the-job drinking, it was hard to believe that he would suddenly get "dog drunk" on the job knowing that he would most likely be caught.

The result: The arbitrator decided that Workman was not drunk, as management claimed, but that he must have consumed some quantity of an alcoholic beverage. The union presented no evidence that the drugs Workman was taking *in themselves* could have caused his symptoms. However, the combination of those drugs with even a small amount of alcohol very likely would have made him appear to be drunk. Reinstatement without back pay was the remedy.[47]

A few more points regarding the "medication defense":

- If an employee drinks even a small amount of alcohol while under medication, he can be held responsible if *the combination of the two adversely affects his ability to do his job.*[48] Normally, however, discharge is too harsh a penalty for such "misconduct," unless he drank enough to be "feeling" it even without the medication.[49]

- Let's say that an employee claims, "It's my medication." The arbitrator agrees: "He's right. There's no evidence of drinking here." Some arbitrators would still penalize the employee even

[47]*United Parcel Service,* 72 LA 1069 (White, 1979). Other "medication defense"-accepted cases include: *Caterpillar Tractor Co.,* 65 LA 159 (Hopson, 1975) (grievant had been given new prescription for his bursitis day before he was reprimanded for being under influence; doctor's note dated shortly thereafter stated that prescription had been too strong and had been discontinued); and *Super Valu Stores, Inc.,* 60 LA 652 (Doyle, 1973) (claim that antihistamines made grievant fall asleep found puzzling, because grievant had not previously told anyone about sinus condition or medication, but proof of intoxication failed because grievant did not appear intoxicated to immediate supervisor).

[48]Although in at least one case the arbitrator placed upon the company the burden of proving that it was the mixture of alcohol and medication and not the medication itself that produced the grievant's symptoms: "It is conceivable, of course, that whatever alcohol T— consumed prior to coming to work interacted with the prescription drugs to produce the behavior noted. However, it is entirely possible that all of the behavior was produced by the drugs, *and the company did not show otherwise.*" (*Caterpillar Tractor Co.,* 65 LA 159, 160 (Hopson, 1975) (emphasis added). In *Park Haven Care Center, Inc.,* 79–2 ARB ¶8328 (Fitzimmons, 1979), the arbitrator reinstated the grievant but imposed a 30-day suspension because she admitted feeling "high" at work from a combination of alcohol and medication.

[49]Where the grievant had between two and four beers and some whiskey during his lunch break, the arbitrator found: "The fact that he may have been taking cold medication which could have enhanced the effects of that alcohol does not excuse the fact that he drank more alcohol than he could handle and was intoxicated upon his return to the plant." (*Baumfolder Corp.,* 78 LA 1060, 1061 (Modjeska, 1982))

though the union argues that a rule prohibiting employees from reporting under the influence of alcohol or drugs should not apply to an employee taking medication prescribed by his physician:

> "To provide such an exception would not be appropriate in my opinion. The purpose of the rule is to safeguard the employee and fellow workers from injury which might occur as a consequence of the employee being under the influence. Whether that influence resulted from the employee taking medication as prescribed or using drugs without benefit of prescription *is not relevant to the fact that the employee was under the influence and therefore a risk in the workplace*"[50] (emphasis added).

- In *FMC Corp.*, the arbitrator suggested that an employee whose capacity to work safely is diminished by medication should take sick leave rather than expose himself and others to hazards at the workplace. *Continental Can Co.* (Example No. 1 above) makes the point that an employee has a *minimum obligation to inform his supervisor* that he is taking drugs that might affect his performance—not only to protect others from potential risks (as *FMC* suggests) but to protect himself from a charge of drunkenness.[51]
- Finally, as a matter of proof, any evidence that directly weakens the company's judgment that an employee was really intoxicated may, by contrast, strengthen the employee's medication defense. For example, in *Park Haven Care Center, Inc.*, 79–2 ARB ¶8328 (Fitzsimmons, 1979), where the evidence against the employee was largely hearsay, the arbitrator rescinded her discharge, concluding:

> "It should also be noted that such things as slurred speech, unsteady gait, glassy eyes and alcoholic odor can be misinterpreted, *particularly when the Grievant has requested the Employer to give her a sobriety test to disprove the existence of intoxication.* This same condition can exist if a person is taking medication, and the person at the same time does have a certain amount of alcohol in her system" (at 4376) (emphasis added).

[50] *FMC Corp.*, 83–1 ARB ¶8324 at 4440 (Reynolds, 1983).

[51] *Super Valu Stores, Inc.*, 60 LA 652, 655 (Doyle, 1973): The grievant "did not indicate to his supervisor at the beginning of his shift that he was not feeling well, and, was not asked, and gave no reason, for wanting a change of duty that night. A prudent person would ordinarily have proffered an explanation of his condition. . . ."

The "illness defense"

ASK YOURSELF:

(The more "Yes" answers, the stronger the defense.)

- Is there corroborating evidence that the employee is really ill, for example:
  - Has he seen a doctor about his condition?
  - Has he recently missed any work days because of illness?
  - Has he previously mentioned his condition to any supervisor, to the company nurse, even to fellow employees?
- Have there been any previous episodes where he has exhibited the same or similar symptoms?
- Does medical opinion confirm that the symptoms of the illness he claims to have are consistent with whatever symptoms led management to believe he was under the influence?
- Is he under any medication that might contribute to his condition? (Obviously the effects of illness and of medication may overlap in some cases.)
- On the whole, is his behavior consistent with being ill rather than being drunk?

A straightforward "illness defense" is less common than a defense based on medication, in part because an employee who is ill often is taking drugs that shift his case over into the "medication" category, and in part because few illnesses produce symptoms similar enough to the symptoms of intoxication to cause confusion. Still, the illness defense does come up, as the following cases illustrate:

EXAMPLE NO. 1: *The superintendent knew and knew he knew*

Harry Workman was found asleep on the job one night and judged by Miles Foreman to be intoxicated; he claimed he had suddenly been overcome by illness and blacked out before he could alert management to the problem. Workman subsequently authorized the company to contact his doctor, who told the superintendent that even though he had not examined Workman up to that point, Workman had called his office to ask for a prescription before the incident. A few days later, after the doctor had examined Workman, he told the superintendent that Workman was suffering from high blood pressure which might cause him to pass out.

As the superintendent was well aware, about two years earlier Workman had collapsed at work after experiencing the same symptoms he experienced on the night in question—indeed, the superintendent had assisted Workman in getting to the hospital on that occasion.

The result: Workman's claim of illness and not being drunk was accepted by the arbitrator. Even though Workman did not see a doctor the day after he blacked out (a fact the arbitrator found surprising), the evidence in Workman's favor was strong enough to outweigh the company's conclusion that he was drunk. The arbitrator faulted the company especially for not asking Workman to take a sobriety test, in view of the fact that the Superintendent was already familiar with his condition and might have determined whether Workman was drunk by that simple expedient.[52]

EXAMPLE NO. 2: *If he doesn't quack like a duck . . .*

Though Workman asked to be excused early because he felt sick, he did not seek medical attention at that time or produce any evidence that he saw a doctor before or after. He did not tell the company the nature of his illness, how long he had been ill, or any other pertinent details. And when confronted by police officers as he sat in his automobile in the company parking lot, he made no response at all when one of the policemen referred to him as "stoned."

The result: Instead of convincing evidence of illness, the arbitrator noted, "we are left with the appearance of a malady of considerable severity which vanished quickly after the close of the shift and required little, if any, more attention from [the grievant.]" Thus, the claim of illness and not being drunk was rejected.[53]

[52]*Kansas-Nebraska Natural Gas Co.;* See KEY CASES IN DETAIL.

[53]*Modern Bakery, Inc.,* 70–2 ARB ¶8599 (Cantor, 1970). In *Evansville State Hospital,* 52 LA 653, 69–2 ARB ¶8585 (Witney, 1969), it was established that the grievant was suffering from a disease of the central nervous system and that either the disease itself or the medication being taken for it could have caused the symptoms which the hospital identified as those of intoxication. However, the grievant had never experienced those symptoms at other times, and the arbitrator found it too coincidental that the single "attack" occurred when the grievant also had alcohol on his breath and admitted to having been drinking the night before. "Illness defense" claims were also rejected in: *General Telephone Co. of California,* 60 LA 1236 (Leventhal, 1973) (though grievant claimed weakness and wobbling were caused by acidosis, he left plant before employer finished making arrangements for him to have doctor check his condition); and *Cal Custom/Hawk,* 65 LA 723 (Ross, 1975) (grievant's belligerent and abusive manner not consistent with depressions).

No less than in medication-defense cases, an employee who claims that what appear to be clear signs of intoxication are really due to illness must produce *credible evidence to support that contention.* The claim "I'm sick!" demands investigation by the company (at least to the extent of questioning the employee to determine whether other evidence can be produced) but an unsupported claim of sickness is not enough to prevent discipline from being imposed.

TAKE THE CASE OF *Tennessee River Pulp & Paper Co.,* 68 LA 421 (Simon, 1976), where the grievant attributed the "weaving or swaying" noticed by supervisors to a six-year-old inner ear problem. The grievant presented no doctor's statement that he had ever been treated and produced no evidence that he had ever been given a prescription for his alleged problem, or that his ears were affected in any way at the time of his discharge. Moreover, he admitted that he had never filed any medical claims, though his medical condition was covered under his employee insurance.

The arbitrator: "[T]hese allegations and/or suggestions regarding *possible* 'ear infection' were completely inadequate to overcome persuasive management testimony that his eyes were red, he smelled strongly of alcohol, his appearance was unkempt, and his speech was slurred and unintelligible—in short, that he was drunk." (at 431)

The "fumes defense"

ASK YOURSELF:

(The more "Yes" answers, the stronger the defense.)

- Have other employees experienced similar problems with the fumes in question?
- Is there medical or scientific evidence that the agent complained of produces the particular effects which the employee exhibits?
- If the employee claims some special sensitivity to the agent, can he substantiate that claim with medical evidence?
- Was the employee present in the area where the fumes are present?

The major problem with the "fumes defense" (and one reason this defense does not figure in as many cases as might be expected) is that toxic chemicals, cleaning agents, and similar products that might give one employee the appearance of being intoxicated probably would affect a number of other employees in the same way. If employees have not generally been affected by fumes, or if no other employees have reported problems, an employee who relies on a fumes defense against charges of intoxication is bound to have a weak case, unless he can prove that he suffers from some special physical sensitivity. By the same token, if fumes present a known problem to employees throughout a department or in the plant, it is the company that may have a difficult case to prove.

SUPPOSE: The happy hour

Harry Workman is discharged after several supervisors decide he is under the influence of alcohol. For 1½ hours, Workman has been working steadily in an area where employees work with solutions containing alcohol and wash out tubs using a thinner containing butyl acetate and other substances. Union officials testify *without contradiction by the company* that the fumes from those agents regularly made employees "sort of happy" so that they had to take breaks outside in the fresh air to clear their heads.

The outcome: Coupled with inconsistent and vague company testimony about Workman's symptoms that night, the strong evidence about the presence of the fumes and their effects persuaded the arbitrator that Workman was not under the influence.[54]

Management v. Union: Which Will Be Believed?

TAKE A HYPOTHETICAL:

Miles Foreman comes to the conclusion that Harry Workman is drunk—he hears him talking loudly to a fellow employee, calling him abusive names; watches him stagger and reach out to the wall for support when he calls him away from his machine; smells whiskey by the time Workman is three or four feet away from him. After he has sent Workman to the personnel office, he questions the three other employees on his crew; they all swear that Harry was *"perfectly all right."*

[54]*The Holliston Mills, Inc.*, 73–1 ARB ¶8177 (Simon, 1973). But in *Okonite Co.*, 74 LA 664 (Ghiz, 1980), the grievant's claim that he was "under the influence" of a cleaning agent failed, even though the chemical was known to cause dizziness and watery eyes, because he had used only a small amount of the product, more than two hours before he was "apprehended," and had had a ready opportunity to have been drinking in the meantime.

If the matter comes before an arbitrator . . . *who will be believed?* There are two factors:

First, the "Shulman connection."[55] For a full discussion of this factor, take a look at "Drinking," Part II below, beginning at p. 94.

Second, quality of testimony. The decision as to who is to be believed—management or union witnesses—also depends on the relative strengths and weaknesses of their respective testimonies.

- *If* a supervisor's report of the employee's behavior is specific and consistent; *if* what he describes matches up with the accepted symptoms of intoxication; *and if* there are no glaring "loopholes" (for example, if the employee had not had the opportunity to drink; or he makes a plausible counterclaim presenting the medication, illness, or fumes defense), the supervisor's judgment that the employee was intoxicated ordinarily will be upheld.
- On the other hand, if a supervisor's credibility is diluted significantly, statements by fellow workers on the employee's behalf will tend to carry more weight. In *The Holliston Mills* case, for example, the contradictory and vague testimony of two supervisors was overwhelmed by employee witnesses' unanimous statements that the grievant showed no signs of being under the influence.[56]
- In order to contribute meaningfully to the grievant's cause, the testimony of union witnesses normally must pass the same credibility tests of specificity, consistency, and so on, that are asked of management witnesses. Thus, where the testimony of several employees that the grievant appeared normal was "somewhat terse and cursory," the arbitrator chose to credit three supervisors whose description of the grievant's condition was, by contrast, "very clear and specific."[57]
- Another reason for crediting the "positive" observations of a supervisor ("I saw X take a drink") over the "negative" evidence offered by employees ("We didn't see X take any drinks") is that the

[55]The volume on Proof contains a detailed discussion of "Shulman connection."

[56]Cited Note 54 above. In *Western Air Lines, Inc.*, 37 LA 130 (Wyckoff, 1961), the arbitrator credited a union witness's testimony that the grievant merely smelled "stale" and was not intoxicated over a supervisor's judgment that she smelled of alcohol, in part because the union witness had a better opportunity to observe the grievant closely and in part because the supervisor was apparently acting on a preconceived notion that an employee who shows up in sunglasses must be trying to conceal evidence of drinking.

[57]*Armstrong Rubber Co.*, 77 LA 775, 778 (Koven, 1981).

employee witnesses may not have been paying sufficient attention to what was there for all to see.[58]

• A fellow employee's *failure* to support the grievant under circumstances where he had a good opportunity to observe his condition weighs heavily against the grievant on the theory that if another employee could honestly have given support, he would have done so.

FOR EXAMPLE:

A missing union witness was a key factor in a case where company security guards accused an employee of reporting to work under the influence. The employee claimed he was not drunk but had become angry and upset only because he believed the guards were hostile because he was black.

The outcome: Because the employee who drove Workman to work that day and witnessed the confrontation was not called to testify, the arbitrator decided management's contention that the grievant was intoxicated had more support.[59]

One final "keep in mind": Even though the supervisor's testimony is believed, and the charge of intoxication is thereby proved, that does not automatically mean that the penalty the company has imposed will be upheld. Appropriateness of penalty is a separate matter from proof of misconduct, as discussed in Chapter 7.

[58]"This of course is a negative: you are more likely to notice something when you are looking for it than when you are busy with something else. . . . Failure to detect is some proof that there is nothing to detect but it is also proof of defective perception or inattention." (*Hughes Air Corp.*, 76–1 ARB ¶8169 (Wyckoff, 1976). A supervisor's positive, credible report cannot be "explained away" in the same manner.

[59]*The Houston Coating Division of AMF Tuboscope, Inc.*, 68–1 ARB ¶8215 (Hon, 1968). "Lukewarm" union testimony on the grievant's behalf can likewise have a damaging effect as, for example, in *Atlantic Steel Co.*, 50 LA 173 (Hebert, 1968), where the arbitrator found unbelievable the testimony of the grievant's brother-in-law that, although he had driven 40 miles to work with the grievant, he did not know whether the grievant had been drinking.

PHYSICAL EVIDENCE

A PREVIEW

- 0.08? 0.10? 0.25? What blood alcohol level proves intoxication?
- Questions of timing
- The "uncorroborated" blood alcohol test
- Where a blood alcohol test helps the most
  - In combination with direct evidence
  - To resolve credibility conflicts
  - To answer "opportunity" questions
- "I object, Mr. Arbitrator!"
  - "That's only hearsay!"
  - Procedural irregularities
  - A little perspective

Physical evidence in a case of suspected intoxication ordinarily refers to blood alcohol tests (more popularly referred to as "sobriety tests") which may be administered either by company medical personnel or at a local hospital or police station. The term "blood alcohol test" has a reassuringly scientific, beyond-a-reasonable-doubt sound to it, and, in contrast to the "subjective" and potentially fallible judgment of a supervisor, it is popularly thought of as an "objective" and accurate standard for deciding whether an employee is intoxicated.

Two important questions concerning "sobriety tests" have already been discussed in Chapter 3, Investigation. To recap briefly, that discussion established that:

- A blood, breath, or urine test is not necessary to prove intoxication (see p. 33); and
- Under many circumstances, if an employee refuses a reasonable request to take a sobriety test, his refusal may be interpreted by an arbitrator as evidence that he is, in fact, under the influence (see p. 35).

In this chapter, the results of sobriety tests come into focus.

0.08? 0.10? 0.25? What Blood Alcohol Level Proves Intoxication?

There are three basic types of "sobriety tests"—drawn blood sample, breath analysis, and urine analysis. All are used to measure the same thing—the quantity of alcohol that an individual has drunk, as indicated by the level of alcohol in his blood.

> "The results of tests for the presence of alcohol in the blood—either by drawn blood sample or by breath or urine analysis—are referred to as the 'Blood Alcohol Concentration' (BAC) and are expressed as a percentage. A result of 0.10 means that alcohol constitutes one-tenth of a percent of the blood serum in the sample. The BAC increases with the number of drinks consumed."[60]

In their most useful chapter on medical evidence in alcohol cases, Denenberg and Denenberg present tables showing the relationship among the amount of 80 proof alcohol consumed on empty and full stomachs, body weight, and BAC. For example, it takes an average of five ounces of 80 proof liquor, consumed on an empty or near-empty stomach, to give a 150-pound individual a BAC of 0.10 percent—the BAC used to define a presumption of "intoxication" in many state motor vehicle codes. Closer to seven ounces would be required to produce the same BAC in a person weighing 200 pounds.[61] But what does a BAC of 0.10 percent really mean?

> *Arbitrator Carnes:* "While it can be depended upon to validly and reliably test blood alcohol content, *individual reactions to a specified level of alcohol in the blood stream cannot be so easily ascertained.*"[62]

A BAC of 0.10 percent or higher is certain evidence that a person has been drinking. But in the absence of behavioral signs of intoxication (staggering, slurring, and the like), it does not *necessarily* prove that he is under the influence to the extent that he cannot function

[60]Denenberg and Denenberg, ALCOHOL AND DRUGS: ISSUES IN THE WORKPLACE (Washington: BNA Books, 1983) pp. 77–78.

[61]To the same effect, in *Tennessee River Pulp & Paper Co.*, 68 LA 421, 427 (Simon, 1976), the arbitrator cited Goodman and Gilman, THE PHARMACOLOGICAL BASIS OF THERAPEUTICS, 2nd edition: "The amount of a particular alcoholic beverage which must be ingested in order to yield a given blood concentration of alchohol varies greatly from person to person and one cannot determine from the blood level the amount of alcohol that was ingested. Conversely, one cannot predict whether the ingestion of a given amount of a particular alcoholic beverage will result in blood levels which are usually associated with intoxication."

[62]*General Felt Industries, Inc.*, 74 LA 972, 976 (1979) (emphasis added).

normally. At very high BAC levels (over 0.20 percent), it is an unusual individual indeed whose mental and physical capacities are not seriously impaired.[63]

At lower levels, however, a person's particular drinking habits may be expected to have a pronounced effect on the amount of alcohol he can consume before feeling or showing any adverse effects. In a leading opinion on this subject, Arbitrator J. A. C. Grant has cited numerous medical studies that show, for example, that a habitually heavy drinker develops a tissue tolerance for alcohol which may require "doses" three to four times greater than a moderate drinker would have to drink to produce characteristic behavioral effects. One physician quoted by Grant notes, "I have seen intoxication . . . with values as low as 0.05%. . . . On the other hand, I have also seen persons with alcohol levels of 0.168%, 0.21%, 0.273% and higher who showed no evidence of intoxication."[64] This is a matter of common experience as well as medical research.

> *Arbitrator Kahn:* "It is well known that people have highly individual tolerances for alcohol. For example, a person who is not accustomed to drinking alcoholic beverages may appear seriously impaired after only an ounce or so. Or, one who drinks just one or two drinks very rapidly, may display all the outward signs of intoxication and yet the blood alcohol test alone—in any of these three illustrations—would not indicate that the blood has a high alcohol content. Conversely, an individual who has been a heavy drinker for a substantial period of time may well develop a much higher tolerance for alcohol, that is, a much greater

[63]"At 0.20 percent . . . the entire motor area of the brain is profoundly affected. The individual tends to assume a horizontal position; he needs help to walk or undress. At 0.30 percent, from the presence of a pint of whiskey in the body . . . the drinker has little comprehension of what he sees, hears or feels; he is stuporous. At 0.40 percent, perception is obliterated; the person is in a coma, he is anesthetized. At 0.60 or 0.70 percent, the lowest, most primitive levels of the brain controlling breathing and heartbeat cease to function and death ensues." (L. Greenberg, "Intoxication and Alcoholism: Physiological Factors," in *Annals of American Academy of Political and Social Science* (January, 1958), 22, 27, cited in Denenberg and Denenberg, Note 60 above.

[64]*Kaiser Steel Corp.*, 31 LA 832, 835 (1958). See also *Tennessee River Pulp & Paper Co.*, 68 LA 421, 427 (Simon, 1976), where a physician consulted by the arbitrator reported that "one person may be *under the influence* when the blood test reveals only 0.05 percent of ethyl alcohol in his blood, while another may have as much as 0.15 percent of ethyl alcohol in his blood and not be *intoxicated*—at that specific moment"; and *Northrop Worldwide Services, Inc.*, 64 LA 742, 749 (Goodstein, 1975), where a physician who testified for the company, when asked if there was any "law" to determine when a person should be arrested for drunk driving, answered: "No, there's no such law because many people are intoxicated, particularly non-drinkers, on a level below that (0.10% or 0.11%) and may be grossly intoxicated."

ability to function well despite large intake. That person, when chemically tested, undoubtedly would show high alcohol level in his blood. Yet even an experienced observer would not detect the signs."[65]

It follows, therefore, is that no single BAC level can be used as sure-fire, "objective" proof of intoxication. That includes BAC levels at which an individual is presumed to be too intoxicated to drive safely under the law.[66]

In one case where the arbitrator decided that the parties must have meant the words "under the influence" in a plant rule to mean under the influence within the meaning of the state's motor vehicle laws (0.10 percent), he still did not accept blood alcohol levels of 0.07 to 0.10 percent and 0.10 to 0.17 percent as proof that the two grievants were intoxicated. Rather, he found that "the objective test results should still be compared against the subjective manifestations."

"The statutory standard," he observed, "has attempted to draw a line at a point where the test itself supplies an accurate reflection of individual capacity, and the judgmental, coordination and physical demands and the safety considerations of operating a motor vehicle are not unrelated to those applicable in a typical factory situation." Statistically speaking, *most* people with a BAC of 0.10% or higher show obvious signs of impairment and are not competent to drive or work safely. The arbitrator continued: "Because the subjective manifestations indicate that [the grievants] were not under the influence at the time they reported to work, I conclude that they would have fallen on the exceptional side of the statistical line. . . . To be sure, they had an alcohol content in their systems. But that of itself is not enough to trigger the rule."[67]

Questions of Timing

TAKE A HYPOTHETICAL:

When Harry Workman reports to work, looking and acting significantly different from normal, Miles Foreman decides that the reason is that he's been drinking. Workman agrees to take a blood test. Four

[65]*Hayes-Albion Corp.*, 76 LA 1005, 1007 (1981).

[66]The arbitrator in *Kaiser Steel*, Note 64 above, quotes numerous sources, including the National Safety Council, as warning that "[t]he results of a chemical analysis should not be the sole criterion upon which an official judgment is based." Denenberg and Denenberg, Note 60 above, also discuss the use of motor vehicle code standards at p. 80ff.

[67]*General Felt Industries, Inc.*, 74 LA 972 (Carnes, 1979).

hours later, when the sample is drawn, his blood alcohol level is 0.055 percent—proof, the union argues vigorously, that Workman was not under the influence as Foreman claimed.

The flaw in the union's not-untypical reasoning is *the time factor.* The effects of alcohol tend to wear off with time. In one case, according to a medical expert on drug and alcohol abuse, alcohol is metabolized by the body at an average rate of 0.02 percent per hour;[68] the figure quoted from another medical source is 0.015 percent per hour.[69]

The slight differences in medical opinion about absorption rates, together with individual differences in how rapidly alcohol is metabolized, make exact backward calculations impossible. But it would still be safe to say in the hypothetical case above that Workman's BAC at the time he reported for work must have been *at least in the neighborhood* of 0.135 percent to 0.115 percent—an estimate which is strongly suggestive of intoxication and which serves to corroborate Foreman's direct evidence.

The "Uncorroborated" Blood Alcohol Test

SUPPOSE: A presumption rebutted?

Shortly after Harry Workman reports for his mid-afternoon shift, Miles Foreman happens to overhear him arguing with another employee—unusual behavior for Workman, who is normally a rather quiet fellow. Foreman challenges Workman for being "under the influence," and Workman denies it. Foreman smells no alcohol at first, but becomes aware of "some smell" when he takes Workman to his office. There is no noticeable staggering.

On his own initiative, Workman gets a blood alcohol test at a local hospital. He is discharged the next day when the company gets the result: a BAC of 0.163 percent, over the legal definition of intoxication under state law (0.10 percent).

Was intoxication proved? "First," the arbitrator pointed out, "the test result merely establishes a presumption that [Workman] was 'under the influence.' *It is a rebuttable presumption, and nothing more.* It does not *prove* that he was so 'under the influence' that he was unable to work."

The more persuasive proof lay in Workman's behavioral symptoms (or lack of them). The only possible symptom of intoxication shown by

[68] *Aerojet Liquid Rocket Co.,* 75 LA 255 (Wollett, 1980). Using that calculation, the expert concluded that since a blood test showed the grievant's blood alcohol level was 0.03% at the time he took the test, it would have been at least 0.10% when he clocked in four hours earlier.

[69] *Cities Service Co.,* 77 LA 1180 (Brisco, 1982).

Workman was his irritability—which, like the alcohol in his system, could have been accounted for by his late partying the night before. Absent greater evidence of impairment, intoxication was not proved.[70]

Thus, even a high BAC level, without corroborating behavioral symptoms, cannot normally be relied upon as proof that an employee is intoxicated. Not only do individuals vary in their tolerance for alcohol, but mistakes can also be made.

A case in point is one where objective evidence from an unbiased source—a lab report placing the employee's BAC at 0.44 percent—was inconsistent with the fact that no one who observed his behavior shortly before the blood sample was drawn noticed any signs of intoxication whatsoever.[71] For the same reasons, a *low* BAC level does not necessarily prove that an employee is *not* under the influence, where direct evidence to the contrary is present.

The "notice exception"

> *Arbitrator Goodstein:* "A blood alcohol test, breath alcohol test or a urine test are all much better criteria [than the opinions of supervisory personnel], *if an alcohol level is set in advance as the point at which the rule is violated or not violated.*"[72]

The one type of case where a particular BAC level, standing alone, stands a good chance of being accepted by an arbitrator as proof of intoxication is that in which the company has put employees on *advance notice* that a specific BAC standard will lead to discipline. Thus, in *Day & Zimmerman,* KEY CASES IN DETAIL, the arbitrator upheld the grievant's discharge in important part because the company demonstrated that *it had consistently used* the level of 0.10% blood alcohol to establish whether an employee was under the influence. In another case the suspension of an employee for working with a BAC of 0.05 percent was upheld where "[l]ong established policy calls for a warning and a work record demerit with a showing of 0.01% on the

[70]*Hayes-Albion Corp.,* 76 LA 1005, 1007 (Kahn, 1981) (emphasis added). In *Kaiser Steel Corp.,* 31 LA 832 (Grant, 1958), the grievant's BAC of 0.19 percent was outweighed by the fact that two physicians who examined him reported no obvious clinical symptoms other than a moderate to slight odor of alcohol; no just cause for discharge.

[71]*Ohio Ferro-Alloys Corp.,* 82–2 ¶8480 (Odom, 1982). The blood sample was taken at a hospital to which the grievant had been admitted for tests and treatment after he fell from an overhead beam in the course of his work.

[72]*Northrop Worldwide Services, Inc.,* 64 LA 742, 749 (1975) (emphasis added).

alcohol blood level test, and suspension or discharge for results showing higher levels of blood alcohol."[73] The message communicated to employees by policies like these is, in effect: If you do *any* drinking before reporting to work, the consequences will be on your own shoulders.[74]

Advance notice that a specific BAC standard will be applied may help the company considerably if it seeks to rely on a blood alcohol test as proof of intoxication. But there are also risks attached to adopting such a specific standard; once the company "picks a number," that's the number it's bound by—whether it likes it or not.

TAKE A LOOK AT:

The Holliston Mills, Inc., 73–1 ARB ¶8177 (Simon, 1973). The grievant's 0.09 percent level of blood alcohol was not accepted as evidence of intoxication where the contract provided that the standard to be applied would be the standard currently accepted by state law enforcement—which was 0.10%.

Where a Blood Alcohol Test Helps the Most

In combination with direct evidence

The results of blood alcohol tests are most useful when they are used to confirm behavioral symptoms of intoxication. In combination with credible direct evidence of intoxication, a test result that shows a significant level of alcohol in the bloodstream makes the conclusion that an employee is under the influence extremely difficult to avoid.

TAKE A LOOK AT:

Aerojet Liquid Rocket Co., 75 LA 256 (Wollett, 1980), where the mutually reinforcing evidence of an objective test and subjective opinion overcame contradictory testimony by the grievant's fellow employees: "Moreover, Dr. Schmidt's testimony with respect to how 0.10 percent alcohol in the bloodstream would manifest itself was corroborated by the observations of supervisors Martynse and Brown and Mr. McLachlan concerning the way F— acted."

[73]*Sperry Rand Corp.*, 59 LA 849, 850 (Logan, 1972).

[74]But in *Northrop Worldwide Services*, cited Note 72 above, the arbitrator refused to uphold the grievant's discharge, even though his blood alcohol level was 0.14 or 0.15 percent, because he had not been told in advance that that BAC would lead to discharge. "In the instant case, there were no criteria at all, but *after the fact*, the Chief decided to set a standard and presented it to the grievant." Likewise *Lockheed Aircraft Corp.*, 28 LA 828, 830 (Hepburn, 1957): "The Company states that a certain percentage of alcohol in the blood constitutes proof of being under the influence of alcohol, and is just cause, but if this meaning has not been communicated to an employee it is not just cause in his case."

> *Tennessee River Pulp & Paper Co.*, 68 LA 421, 431 (Simm, 1976). "In view of the admissibility of the blood alcohol test which conclusively proved that the Grievant was at least *under the influence* of alcohol. . . ; and, in view of the obvious recognition by four members of management that he appeared to be intoxicated, your Arbitrator must uphold the Company's contention that it had proper and just 'cause' to suspend and later discharge the Grievant. . . ."
>
> *Day & Zimmerman, Inc.*, 75 LA 699, 701 (Sisk, 1980). "The investigation prior to G—'s discharge was complete in every respect. There was the observation of his immediate superintendent. That observation is verified by the objective findings of the breathalyzer test."[75]

To resolve credibility conflicts

Because the blood alcohol test provides an accurate measurement of the minimum amount of alcohol consumed, it can function in many situations as a test of an employee's credibility.

"I just had two beers!" Or so the grievant often claims. But "unless the glasses were bucket sized," the arbitrator found in one case, the grievant's 0.19 percent blood alcohol level established that he had had a lot more than that—eight ounces of whiskey would have been more like it.[76] In another case, the grievant claimed that his BAC of 0.215 percent was explained by four beers, consumed 12 hours before a blood sample was drawn. That claim was rejected as "fantastic" by the arbitrator.[77]

When an employee's credibility is punctured *on a specific point* such as how much he had to drink, his credibility *as a whole* often becomes suspect.

> *Arbitrator Brisco:* "Whatever the exact time, it is medically impossible for two beers to result some nine to 11 hours later in a blood alcohol level of 0.46%. The grievant's testimony on this point is so egregiously false that the Arbitrator has been forced to give little weight to her other testimony where it conflicts with the observations of . . . credible percipient witnesses to [her] behavior after she reported for work."[78]

[75]Also *Sperry Rand Corp.*, Note 73 above ("W—clocked in two hours and twenty-four minutes late; he evidenced unusual conduct and behavior; a test to determine the blood levels of alcohol in his system . . . showed an alcohol blood level of 0.05%."); and *Alameda-Contra Costa Transit District*, 80–1 ARB ¶8060, 3275 (Randall, 1979) ("The observations of the four percipient witnesses, without more, are convincing evidence that Grievant was under the influence. . . . The blood test may thus be viewed as merely corroborative.")

[76]*Kaiser Steel Corp.*, 31 LA 832 (J. A. C. Grant, 1958).

[77]*Tennessee River Pulp & Paper Co.*, 68 LA 421 (Simon, 1976).

[78]*Cities Service Co.*, 77 LA 1181, 1182–3 (1982).

"It's my medication!" Whether an employee's unusual behavior is really due to alcohol or to some more "innocent" cause can many times be resolved definitively by means of a blood alcohol test. Where test results give evidence of drinking, the medication (or illness or fumes) defense will be difficult for an employee to sustain.[79]

To answer "opportunity" questions

A blood alcohol test can sometimes pinpoint when an employee did his drinking, where opportunity is a crucial question.

SUPPOSE: *No other explanation*

When Harry Workman clocks in at about 2:15 P.M., he appears to be fit to work, though one supervisor notices the smell of alcohol on his breath. About an hour later, however, his work habits become erratic and he burns himself as a result. The employer concludes that he must have been intoxicated and fires him under a rule that makes discharge the penalty for a first offense of having intoxicants in his possession on company property.

The union contends that Workman was not drinking on company premises, but he had had a few drinks at home that morning—so that, *at worst,* he should have been disciplined under a different rule making suspension the penalty for reporting under the influence.

The deciding factor: A blood alcohol test showed Workman's BAC at 4:00 P.M. to have been 0.26 percent—too high to be accounted for by any preshift imbibing, in view of the fact that he did not seem obviously intoxicated to two supervisors who saw him shortly thereafter. The discovery of an almost-empty whiskey bottle in his locker clinched the company's case—discharge was sustained.[80]

[79]"It becomes difficult for an employer to sustain an allegation of . . . drinking when faced with conflicting testimony and the existence of another probable cause for an employee's [unusual] behavior. The employer's safest course of action under most circumstances is to obtain competent medical verification when an employee's condition is suspect. Similarly, if the employee's defense . . . is the existence of an alternative medical condition, . . . he too is safest in having the matter determined by competent medical authority." (*General Telephone Co. of Calif.*, 60 LA 1236, 1238 (Leventhal, 1973) The importance of getting a confirming blood alcohol test where an illness is in issue was also stressed by the arbitrator in *Kansas-Nebraska Natural Gas Co.*, KEY CASES IN DETAIL.

[80]*Atlantic Steel Co.*, 50 LA 173 (Hebert, 1968). The grievant's high BAC also disproved the grievant's claim that he had been drinking before work, and not on company premises during his lunch break in *Beatrice Foods*, 73 LA 191 (Thornell, 1979).

"I object, Mr. Arbitrator—that's only hearsay!"

> Hearsay is testimony given (or a statement made) by a person who reports not what he knows, but what he has heard from someone else, for the purpose of proving the truth of the matter stated.

In the great majority of arbitration cases, blood alcohol test results are admitted into evidence and credited by the arbitrator as a routine matter (with the understanding that what those results mean may be a matter of argument). However, in the case of *Alameda-Contra Costa Transit District,* 80–1 ARB ¶8060 (Randall, 1979), the employer found that its offer of a lab report met with determined opposition from the union on the following grounds:

First: Blood alcohol test results are hearsay and therefore inadmissible. A statement on a laboratory report that Grievant X's blood alcohol level was 0.20 percent is hearsay in the sense that the employer has no direct, personal knowledge of the truth of that report. For example, the employer cannot state of his own knowledge that the blood tested really came from the grievant and that the grievant's name did not somehow get on someone else's sample. He cannot state that correct testing procedures were observed in the lab. He cannot state that a typographical error was not made in the report itself, and that "0.20" could not have been "0.10."

Second, the "business records" exception to the hearsay rule does not apply. A blood alcohol test report is not a business record because it is prepared in contemplation of disciplinary action, and not in the regular course of the hospital's business or as part of the grievant's medical treatment.

Third, the strict foundational requirements that the courts impose for the admission of tests results were not met. Those requirements include, e.g., that the "prosecution" prove through *witnesses* to the blood sampling and analyzing process that blood taken from the grievant was the blood tested; that the needle and syringe were sterile; that alcohol was not used as a disinfectant; that the laboratory equipment was working properly.

Fourth, the blood sample was not preserved and made available to grievant. Even the most reliable scientific test is subject to human error, and the grievant's due process right to material which might have helped him was violated when he was denied the opportunity to "cross-examine" the blood sample by independent testing.

The arbitrator rejected the union's objections on the ground that the lab report did, in fact, qualify as a business record. He found further that the employer had laid an adequate foundation for the admission of the test results into evidence.[81]

> "(a) *The test results were made in the regular course of Herrick's [the hospital's] business.* (Had the District conducted the test itself, this would not be so; the results would be "in contemplation of litigation" and therefore inadmissible. But the conduct of the test was routine business insofar as Herrick was concerned; it apparently did not even know the purpose for which the results were sought.)
>
> "(b) *The writings (labeling of the sample, recording of the test results) were made at or near the time of the event (drawing of the sample, completing of the test).* Herrick's standard procedure is for a sample to be labeled with the subject's name at the time it is drawn, while the individual is still present. Test results are recorded upon completion of the test procedure.
>
> "(c) *The writings were identified and their mode of preparation were described by a qualified witness (technologist [C]).*
>
> "(d) *The sources of information and method and time of preparation were such as to indicate its trustworthiness.* The sample in question was tested approximately an hour after it was drawn. Since Herrick is a neutral party, there is no reason to suspect that the sample was deliberately tampered with. The test was conducted by medical technologist [C], who described her procedure in detail at the hearing."

The arbitrator also decided that the test results should not be disregarded just because the blood sample itself was destroyed, since it was not destroyed in bad faith.

Procedural Irregularities

Objection may also be raised to the admission and consideration of blood alcohol test results if there were any irregularities in administering the test or handling the physical evidence. Where irregularities are serious enough to have possibly compromised the test's accuracy, the results may well be disregarded by the arbitrator.

[81]Section 1271 of the California Evidence code cited as follows: "Evidence of a writing made as a record of an act, condition, or event is not made inadmissible by the hearsay rule when offered to prove the act, condition or event if: (a) The writing was made in the regular course of a business: (b) the writing was made at or near the time of the act, condition, or event; (c) the custodian or other qualified witness testifies to its identity and the mode of its preparation; and (d) the sources of information and method and time of preparation were such as to indicate its trustworthiness.

A Little Perspective

• For the most part, technical rules of evidence are not observed in arbitration. Most arbitrators would admit hearsay evidence, even if only "for the weight it deserves," so that blood test results can make their way into the record on that basis alone. Even for arbitrators who are "tough" on hearsay, the business-records exception to the hearsay rule ordinarily justifies the admission of test results.

• *Proof* that a blood alcohol test was mishandled in some way is required if the arbitrator is to reject the test results. The *possibility* of irregularity or error is ordinarily not enough, although the weight which the arbitrator might otherwise have attached to a blood alcohol test in *The Holliston Mills, Inc.,* 73–1 ARB ¶8177 (Simon, 1973) was considerably reduced because a supervisor, instead of mailing the grievant's blood sample to a toxicology laboratory in the presence of a union official, left it in a box at the plant with other outgoing mail, where anyone could have tampered with it.

• Even though test results are the product of hearsay, they become less vulnerable to attack for that reason when they have some testimonial foundation, e.g., testimony (subject to cross-examination, of course) of the particular technician who actually conducted the test.

• Objections to the admission and consideration of test results carry greatest weight when the results are clearly in conflict with other evidence. For example, in *Ohio Ferro-Alloys Corp.,* 82–2 ARB ¶8480, 5156 (Odom, 1982), a lab report which stated that the grievant was working with a BAC of 0.44 percent failed to persuade the arbitrator that the grievant was intoxicated. The grievant showed no behavioral symptoms of intoxication whatsoever, and "no one who had even seen the blood, much less handled it, testified with regard to the care taken in performing the test and the conditions prevailing in the laboratory."

• On the other side of the coin, even real and substantial questions about the reliability of a lab report lose their "punch" when persuasive direct evidence of intoxication is present. In *Alameda-Contra Costa,* the arbitrator noted, "[f]or purposes of this arbitration, there is also a special factor weighing in favor of admissibility, *even if the degree of accuracy of the test is questionable.* That is, it is of no import whether Grievant had *exactly* a 0.25 percent blood level." (at 3273) Four employer witnesses testified credibly that the grievant was under the influence, and even a convincing showing by the union that the test could have been "off" by as much as 150 percent could not dilute the effect of that testimony.

CHECKLIST—ASK YOURSELF:

(The more "Yes" answers, the more persuasive the proof of intoxication.)

Direct Evidence

- Are all (or at least a substantial number of) the accepted symptoms of intoxication present?
- Is the credibility of the company's case undiluted by any of the following problems:
  - The "single symptom" problem?
  - Key symptom missing?
  - Delayed reaction?
  - The "opportunity factor"?
  - Conflicting, inconsistent, vague, and otherwise incredible testimony?
  - Hearsay?
- If the employee has put forward one of the "three classic defenses" against intoxication charges, has his defense been successfully ruled out?
  - The "medication defense"?
  - The "illness defense"?
  - The "fumes defense"?
- Investigation
  - Did the employee refuse to take a blood alcohol test, without having a legitimate reason for his refusal?
  - If the employee volunteered to take a blood alcohol test, did the company agree to his request? (If he was not given that opportunity when he asked for it, an inference might be drawn that he was sober and knew it.)

Physical Evidence

- *Corroboration:* Are blood alcohol test results corroborated by direct evidence of intoxication?

- *Credibility questions:* Is the employee's blood alcohol level high enough to support the company's theory that he was intoxicated? (Rather than low enough to support the grievant's disclaimer—"I only had two beers.")
- *The "opportunity factor":* Does the employee's blood alcohol level tend to confirm the company's theory that he must have been drinking at work or immediately before work? (Rather than support the employee's story—"I haven't had a drop since that party last night.")
- *Hearsay:* Can the company lay an adequate foundation for introducing blood alcohol test results—e.g., by producing a witness to testify about the laboratory's procedures—if the case goes to arbitration, and the union challenges the lab report as "hearsay"?
- *Procedural problems:* Was the administration of the blood alcohol test free from procedural irregularities?
- *"Notice":* If a particular blood alcohol percentage is relied upon as the only (or even as the primary) evidence that the employee was under the influence, did the company put employees on advance notice that the standard would be applied?

II. DRINKING

DRINKING V. INTOXICATION: TWO DIFFERENT PROBLEMS OF PROOF

Proof of drinking differs from proof of intoxication in two critical respects. *First,* convincing evidence that an employee is intoxicated may indicate that he has been drinking at work; but if an employee has not yet been drinking to the point where he is under the influence, there may be no physical signs at all—other than, in some cases, the smell of alcohol on the breath. *Second,* while proof of intoxication is almost invariably based on direct evidence, sometimes in combination with medical test results, drinking may be proved in *either one of two ways,* depending on the facts of the case.

PROOF OF DRINKING: A PREVIEW

Typically, evidence that an employee has been drinking on the job falls into one of two basic categories:

1. *Direct evidence*—a supervisor's statement like "I saw him do it," which may or may not be supported by other facts; or
2. *Circumstantial evidence*—that "chain of circumstances" which leads to the conclusion that the employee must have been drinking.

DIRECT EVIDENCE

Credibility is the key to direct evidence. In drinking cases, the typical and most frequent confrontation takes place between a supervisor (or security guard or watchman) who says he saw an employee take a drink and the employee who says he did not. The problem is therefore simple enough to state—*who is to be believed.* But usually it is not so simple to decide.

Five Crucial Questions

A supervisor or other company witness can test his own credibility in a drinking case by asking himself the following questions:

ASK YOURSELF:

("Yes" answers down the line add up to strong evidence of drinking. But too many "No" answers could scuttle the employer's case before an arbitrator—even when the supervisor knows in his heart that he is right.)

1. Did the supervisor have a clear view of what the employee was doing?

2. Was he sure of what he saw— certain about the identity of the employee?
3. Was he sure that what the employee was drinking was alcohol?
4. Did the supervisor locate any corroborating evidence, such as a liquor bottle or beer can—empty or not?
5. Did the supervisor conduct a thorough investigation?

Take a look at the following four examples of how these questions can become crucial problems of proof for the company.

BEER, OR JUST SODA?—THE "CLEAR VIEW" QUESTION

Three employees are spotted by supervisors drinking beer in the company parking lot during their break. The employees later claim that they were only drinking soft drinks. The company is skeptical, and discharges them.

The problem: In a reenactment of the scene under similar lighting conditions, the same supervisors could not distinguish between beer cans and soda cans from the same rooftop vantage point, even though one supervisor had previously identified the cans as a particular *brand* of beer. Concluding that the supervisors could not have been sure just what they saw on the night in question, the arbitrator overturned the discharges.[82]

THE "WHAT WAS IT?," "WHO WAS IT?" QUESTION

The union claims "mistaken identity" when Harry Workman is discharged for taking a drink by Dave Powers, the new branch manager who had only been there a short time. As for the liquid Powers saw Workman consume—only grapefruit juice, the union says.

The time, the company fares better. On the "Who was it?" question, Powers made sure of his identification by pointing Workman out within a few minutes to another supervisor who knew Workman by name. Moreover, only four other employees were present in the department at the time, so the chances of mistaken identity were slight.

[82] *W. R. Grace & Co.*, 69 LA 1071 (Flaten, 1977).

The union's challenge on the "What was it?" issue also fails. Powers retrieved the cup immediately after Workman discarded it, determined by the smell that it had contained liquor and had two other supervisors immediately smell it. They too were positive it had contained alcohol.[83]

FIND THE BODY—THE "CORROBORATING EVIDENCE" QUESTION

Miles Foreman and Andy King both state that they saw Harry Workman and Alan Alpha drinking beer in the parking lot. Workman and Alpha swear, however, that they found beer bottles under the tires of a car and were throwing them away—not drinking from them.

What decided this case? Two facts are pivotal: that the security guard who investigated the incident reported no smell of beer at the scene and that he failed to recover the beer bottles from the trash to see if they were still cold and wet or if in any way they showed they had been recently drunk from. Without that key evidence, the arbitrator had to conclude that the grievants might have been telling the truth.[84]

"OUT TO LUNCH"—THE "THOROUGH INVESTIGATION" QUESTION

Workman is observed by Miles Foreman taking a drink from a whiskey bottle and throwing the empty bottle away. To reach the scene, some 50 feet away, Foreman has to take a roundabout route, and by the time he reaches the area Workman has left by another exit for his meal break. When Workman returns, he denies having taken a drink.

Where Foreman blew his chance: He retrieved the bottle, but, by waiting to confront Workman until after he had finished his meal instead of immediately going after him, he lost the chance to find out for sure

[83]*Duchess Furniture Co.*, 74–1 ARB ¶8276 (King, 1974). In *Cessna Aircraft Co.*, 52 LA 764 (Altrock, 1969), the arbitrator rejected the union's argument that the foreman could not be *certain* the grievant was drinking—even though he saw him raise a cup, which was found to contain alcohol, to his lips. "How in the world," the arbitrator asked, "does one tell whether a man is actually swallowing?" He took a "common sense" view and decided that the grievant did drink from the liquid in the cup. Under some circumstances, however, arbitrators have been more skeptical; see *St. Louis Diecasting Corp.*, cited below ("Out to Lunch").

[84]*Dayton Press, Inc.*, 80–1 ARB ¶8210 (Thomson, 1980). The fact that no liquor, bottles, or beer cans were reported to have been on the scene where the grievant was supposedly seen drinking helped convince the arbitrator of his innocence in *Chicago Transit Authority*, 77–2 ARB ¶8375 (Larkin, 1977); evidence that the accusing supervisor had earlier threatened to "get his job" was another factor.

if Workman had been drinking. Food probably would have erased any liquor smell from Workman's breath, so that being able to provide satisfactory proof became all but impossible.[85]

The "Shulman Connection"

In its distilled form, the "Shulman connection" goes something like this:

• Harry Workman says, "I didn't do it." Miles Foreman says, "Yes, you did. I saw you do it."

• Both witnesses testify in a straightforward manner. Both seem to be telling the truth. There is no evidence of any trouble between the two men—no showing of bias, malice, jealousy; only a business-like, reserved, what might be described as a "friendly" employment relationship.

• Both testify at the grievance steps, and the story each tells is consistent with what he testifies to at the arbitration. No facts disprove or contradict their respective versions.

• No other witnesses testify.

And so who is to prevail—Miles Foreman or Harry Workman? The "Shulman connection" says you simply credit Miles Foreman (or the accuser, as the case may be): "An accused employee is presumed to have an incentive for not telling the truth and that when his testimony is contradicted by one who has nothing to lose or gain, the latter is to be believed."[86]

[85]*St. Louis Diecasting Corp.*, 69–1 ARB ¶8163 (Erbs, 1968). In large measure because of the supervisor's failure to follow up his investigation promptly, the arbitrator also had to question what the supervisor "really saw." He believed the supervisor's story that the grievant raised the bottle to his lips and that the supervisor smelled whiskey when he retrieved the bottle from the trash can. But he decided that, at a distance of 50 feet, the supervisor could not have been certain that there was anything *in* the bottle when the grievant raised it to his lips. Only the grievant would know; and he denied the whole incident. And the supervisor missed the opportunity to get the remaining evidence, i.e., the odor on the grievant's breath.

The company also bungled its investigation in *W. R. Grace & Co.*, Note 82 above. After the three grievants were seen allegedly drinking beer, the plant manager went down and told them all to go home—without telling them why. He noticed at that time that one employee had a can tucked into his jacket, but did not ask what it was or ask to see it. Nor did he, or anyone else from the company, try to retrieve the cans from where the employees were seen to have dropped them.

[86]*Ford Motor Co.*, 1 ALAA 67,244 (1945); 1 ALAA 67,620 (1954). Cited variously throughout cases and in arbitration literature, e.g., Stessin, EMPLOYEE DISCIPLINE (Washington: BNA Books, 1961), p. 44; *United Parcel Service, Inc.*, 66–2 ARB ¶8703, at 5432 (Dolson, 1966); *Western Condensing Co.*, 37 LA 912, 914 (Mueller, 1962); *Riley-Stoker Co.*, 63 LA 581, 584, 74–2 ARB ¶8434, (Shister, 1974); *Motor Transportation Co.*, 76 LA 958, 960 (Talent, 1981).

Why is Miles Foreman entitled to be credited over Harry Workman? Because Harry Workman has an *interest* to protect—namely his job.[87] Such an interest "is cause for suspicion and tends to weaken credibility,"[88] because "when an employee's job is at stake, his testimony is generally an exercise in self-absolution."[89] Thus under the "Shulman connection," Miles Foreman, and not Harry Workman, would tend to be credited *if* he satisfies most—not necessarily all—of the following conditions:[90]

- IF—Miles Foreman has nothing immediately to gain or to lose in the case;
- IF—Foreman had no reason to single out Harry Workman;
- IF—there is no reason to conclude that Foreman was mistaken;
- IF—there is no evidence of bad feeling or ill will (or bias, malice, prejudice, discrimination, jealousy, hostility, anger, etc.) toward Harry Workman;
- IF—on its face, Miles Foreman's story is not incredible;
- IF—Miles Foreman is a long-service employee and Harry Workman is a relatively new employee, the "Shulman connection" is particularly favored.[91]

[87]*Campbell Industries,* 72–1 ARB ¶8120 (Block, 1972).

[88]Richard Mittenthal, "Credibility—A Will-o'-the-Wisp," in TRUTH, LIE DETECTORS, AND OTHER PROBLEMS IN LABOR ARBITRATION. Proceedings of the 31st Annual Meeting, National Academy of Arbitrators (Washington, D.C.: BNA Books, 1979), p. 68.

[89]*Kraft Foods, Inc.,* 73 LA 493 (Rose, 1979). For reasoning that goes beyond the Shulman rationale in preferring supervisor over grievant testimony, see *Standard Oil Co. (Indiana),* 19 LA 795 (Naggi, 1952): "To rule against management in a case based solely on the personal testimony of a member of the supervision staff as against the personal testimony of two employees could very well, in the future, jeopardize the responsibility vested in those who direct and supervise." Naggi sees the position of the supervisor as identical to that of a law enforcement official: "As effectively stated by the Company," he says, "the position of the supervisor in the apprehension of violators of Company regulations is analogous to that of law enforcement agencies in which the police officers report of the incident as observed by him is acknowledged to be valid evidence." In passing it should be observed that Naggi's notion has not caught on well; for the view that supervisors are human and can be mistaken, see *U.S. Industrial Chemicals Co.,* 77–1 ARB ¶8084 (Edelman, 1977).

[90]*Ford Motor Co.,* Note 86 above. In general accord, *American Motors,* 69–2 ARB ¶8504, 52 LA 709 (Keefe, 1969); *Pennsylvia Greyhound Lines, Inc.,* 19 LA 210 (Seward, 1952); *Sun Shipbuilding & Drydock Co.,* 1 ALAA 67,648 (1947). Also see *General Electric Co.,* 40 LA 1084 (Crawford, 1963); *Hawaiian Airlines, Inc.,* 70–2 ARB ¶8563 (Tsukiyama, 1970); *Lake Orion Community Schools,* 73 LA 707 (Roumell, 1979); *Grand Union Co.,* 48 LA 812 (Scheiber, 1967); *Billingsley, Inc.,* 48 LA 802 (Krimsly, 1967). *St. Louis Diecasting Corp.,* 69–1 ARB ¶8163 (Erbs, 1968).

[91]Owen Fairweather, PRACTICE AND PROCEDURE IN LABOR ARBITRATION (Washington, D.C.: BNA Books, 1973), pp. 216–17. Cited in a number of cases including the key case of *Babcock & Wilcox Co.,* 74–1 ARB ¶8223 (Geissinger, 1974), and *Motor Transportation Co.,* 76 LA 958 (Talent, 1981).

NOTE ALSO that arbitrators generally require that a union corroborate its interested witnesses' testimony when it is in conflict with the testimony of management witnesses.

Let's say that a supervisor can confidently answer "Yes" to all five "crucial questions." He hasn't done any of the things that would put him in an unfavorable light—e.g., jumping to conclusions or letting evidence slip through his fingers. In his own mind, he's absolutely certain that he saw an employee take a drink. If the employee continues to deny it, who will be believed?

TAKE A TYPICAL CONFRONTATION

The facts: During their lunch break, Harry Workman and Mike Armstrong drive in Armstrong's car to a shopping center, about a half mile from the plant, where Workman purchases a six-pack of beer. The two men return to the company parking lot. Workman gets out of the car, takes the six-pack—which now contains only five full cans of beer—to his own car, and throws an empty can on the ground.

Security guard Dick Sargent is on the scene in the parking lot. *According to Sargent,* as Workman got out of Armstrong's car, just before he threw away the can, he tipped the can to his mouth and consumed the remaining contents. *Workman claims,* on the other hand, that he drank the full can of beer while he was still at the shopping center and did not consume a drop on company premises.

Investigation: Neither the union nor the company can produce any witness to corroborate Workman's or Sargent's story. The empty can is retrieved from the ground and the five full cans are confiscated. An examination of Armstrong's car reveals 13 other empty beer cans which are also confiscated.

What the arbitrator was faced with was a classic case of one man's word against the other's—with no "hard" evidence to support either one. The arbitrator reasoned as follows:

"[The guard] is presumed to be a trained Security Officer, with such training including the ability to be highly observant. Further, [the guard's] position presumes that he has a function to perform—often controversial—but *one that gains him no favor for and includes no need to engage in falsification.*

"*The potential advantages to [the grievant] to dispute [the guard's] testimony are self-evident in this case,* and the tendency of an employee to do so under the circumstances is understandable."

The conclusion: the company proved its case that the grievant was drinking on company property and discharge was sustained.[92]

Picking on Shulman

The "Shulman connection" has its critics among arbitrators (and understandably even more so among union people). An anti-Shulman view usually starts with the proposition that "[a] witness should not be discredited because he has a bias or interest in the matter about which he testified"[93] (and, conversely, "[a] witness should not be considered truthful merely because he has no bias or interest in the matter about which he testified"[94]). In other words, self-interest "does not impeach a witness' credibility by and of itself,"[95] and "an interest in the outcome does not raise any presumption that a discharged employee is lying."[96]

It is next pointed out that while Miles Foreman may not have had an "interest" to start with, now that the matter has been grieved he surely has an "interest in the outcome" because he wants his discharge of Harry to be validated. Thus, both Harry Workman and Miles Foreman have an "interest in the outcome," although the character of their respective "interests" may differ.[97] At rock-bottom, say these critics, each man very much wants to win.

[92]*AMF Lawn & Garden Div.,* 64 LA 988 (Wyman, 1975).

[93]Mittenthal, Note 88 above, at 68.

[94]*Id.* at 68–69.

[95]*Texas Mills Supply & Mfg. Co.,* 74–2 ARB ¶8703 (Marlatt, 1975) goes on to state: "One must determine whether the testimony is inconsistent, contrary to known facts, or inherently improbable."

[96]*Billingsley, Inc.,* Note 90 above: "I will first state that interest in the outcome as a factor to consider in biased testimony is a far cry from the assumption that the grievant is lying or presenting a gross distortion. . . . If the grievant's testimony is colored by bias, it must be remembered that the Company's witness, all employees, are also considered having a bias by reason of their employment requiring close scrutiny; however, nothing in either of those relationships to a matter in arbitration can be taken to mean there is any presumption any witness shall lie." (at 807) See also *Community Warehouse Corp.,* 60 LA 1260, 1264 (Doppelt, 1973): "While it is true that grievant has a greater self-interest . . . than L—, it should not lightly be presumed that he is lying. A man is presumed innocent from the outset, and a person will deny a theft because of his true innocence as well as from self-interest. It is just as fair to presume that grievant denied his complicity in the theft because he was innocent thereof, as it is to presume that he perjured himself out of self-interest."

[97]Moreover, some supervisors, especially new ones, "could be open to a charge of interest, in seeking to curry management's favor." *Alcolac Chemical Corp.,* 55 LA 306, 311 (Robertson, 1970).

"The argument that the testimony of the Union's witnesses is to be disregarded because 'all of the witnesses are prejudiced, since they are members of the Union and/or officers of the local Lodge,' combined with the assertion . . . that the testimony of a supervisor is to be accepted implicitly because 'He has no axe to grind' is unacceptable either as good law or good labor relations.

"The expected bias of parties in interest does not disqualify them as witnesses."[98]

Those who make a frontal attack upon the "Shulman connection" usually emphasize that it is out of synch with three fundamental, time-honored, and controlling principles, namely, the burden of proof (which is, of course, the employer's to bear)[99] and its supporting buttresses—"the benefit of the doubt" (in favor of the grievant)[100] and "the presumption of innocence" (also in favor of the grievant).[101] In addition, a number of other criticisms of Shulman have been lodged: that the "Shulman connection" is dependent upon an "upper-class bias" (Ben Fischer of the United Steelworkers);[102] that supervisors are human and can be mistaken;[103] that the "Shulman connection" as such should be shelved, and that one can more profitably look elsewhere, e.g., to the testimony as a whole and whether the employer's conduct was based on "substantial evidence."[104] Finally there is what might be called the "Mittenthal variations."

The "Mittenthal variations:" Without naming Shulman specifically by name, Arbitrator Richard Mittenthal essentially has proposed a modification of the "Shulman connection" in which he seeks to retain

[98]*Poloron Products of Pa., Inc.*, 23 LA 789 (Rosenfarb, 1955): "Being human, both sides might be subject to the unconscious influence of self-interest, personal predilection or antipathy. It is the province and the duty of the one making the decision not to engage in all-encompassing, invariable generalities, but to examine the testimony of each witness on its own merits."

[99]*FMC Corporation,* 73 LA 705 (Marlatt, 1979).

[100]*Giant Food, Inc.*, 72 LA 281 (Fields, 1979).

[101]*Standard Oil of Ohio.*, 75 LA 588 (Kindig, 1980). Of course, if the grievant's own credibility is punctured in any significant way, then the "presumption of innocence" would be lost and a supervisor who testifies credibly and consistently could be expected to prevail. In *AMF Lawn & Garden Div.,* Note 92 above, the company's case gained additional strength from the dubious nature of the grievant's explanation: "[H]is testimony that he held an empty beer can in his hand for the one-half mile distance from the shopping center parking lot to the Company's parking lot seems incongruous. To do so, in the back of a vehicle containing 13 other empty beer cans, seems to violate normal behavior—which would have been to deposit the empty can among the others rather than to have departed from the vehicle and deposited it on the parking lot ground."

[102]*National Food Stores of Louisiana, Inc.*, 74–2 ARB ¶8512 (Marlatt, 1974).

[103]*U.S. Industrial Chemicals Co.*, 77–1 ARB ¶8084 (Edelman, 1977).

[104]*Parkview-Gem Inc.*, 59 LA 429 (Dugan, 1972); *Kroger Co.,* 68–2 ARB ¶8787, 5736, 51 LA 251 (Scheib, 1968).

its core and at the same time satisfy some of the objections previously mentioned. Here is the modification in Mittenthal's words:

> "First, the employee who denies wrongdoing has a clear interest in avoiding punishment. That interest, by itself, is no basis for discrediting his testimony. But it does serve to weaken his credibility just as the foreman's lack of interest serves to strengthen his credibility. The real issue thus becomes one of *relative credibility* (emphasis added). Only if the foreman's credibility is substantially greater than the employee's should management win. Inteest alone may tilt the scales in some cases but not in others. There are, after all, a myriad of factors to be evaluated in each dispute. Not the least of them is the arbitrator's own intuitions, his feelings about the evidence, the arguments, and the texture of the case. What must be avoided is an uncritical adoption of interest as a decisive factor in the close case, for that would mean that the foreman's accusation would always prevail over the employee's denial."[105]

Hearsay Evidence

The dubious value of hearsay as evidence on which to base disciplinary action has already been mentioned in the context of proving intoxication (see p. 65 above). Hearsay may put in an appearance in cases of simple drinking as well. This often occurs where an employee's drinking comes to the company's attention through the report of a security officer, watchman, or other individual. When the case comes to arbitration, if the report is the only evidence put forward that the employee was drinking—and if the person who made the report does not appear to testify—any testimony offered about the report normally will be given little weight because of its *hearsay character*. The following example illustrates why.

SUPPOSE: *Reports and dead men tell no tales*

The company receives a written report from a security guard that he saw Harry Workman in the parking lot drinking from a can of beer. Upon investigation, a half-full beer can and a bag of empties are found in Workman's work area, and he is discharged as a result.

The catch: Another employee, Mike Armstrong, was with Workman in the parking lot that night, and Workman testifies that it was

[105]Mittenthal, Note 88 above, at 70. See also *American Trailers, Inc.*, 73–2 ARB ¶8348 (Merrill, 1973), where the grievant did not directly deny the charge that he had been drinking until the arbitration hearing, and *Pacific Telephone & Telegraph Co.*, 56 LA 1191 (Hughes, 1971), where reasons not to credit the grievant's testimony included self-interest; a record of prior misconduct; self-contradictions within his own story; and evidence that he had used force and threats on his accuser (a company customer) to persuade her to change her testimony.

Armstrong who was doing the drinking. The light was bad and the guard was about 100 feet away from the "phantom drinker." How, then, could the guard be so sure it was Workman and not Armstrong that he saw? The guard's written report did not answer that question, and neither did the guard—since by the time the arbitration rolled around he had already left the state and did not testify.

The outcome: The arbitrator found that the report not only was strictly hearsay, it was open to question even on its face—and could not serve as adequate proof that Workman had been drinking.[106]

A general rule of thumb: Only where hearsay is introduced *together with* other convincing evidence that an employee was drinking is hearsay likely to have an impact on an arbitrator's decision.[107]

CIRCUMSTANTIAL EVIDENCE

Arbitrator Jacobs: "Grievant was discharged for drinking on the job. He was not discharged for allegedly being intoxicated while on the job.

"This distinction is important in view of the fact that the evidence in support of the allegation is, as was admitted by the Company, largely circumstantial evidence. While it would be extremely difficult, if not in fact impossible to prove intoxication by circumstantial evidence, the allegation of drinking on the job may be proved by circumstantial evidence." (*McCormick & Baxter Creosoting Co.;* see KEY CASES IN DETAIL)

Contrary to what the union sometimes argues, the company does not necessarily have to come up with direct evidence—the "I saw with

[106]*Anvan Industries, Inc.*, 72–2 ARB ¶8516 (Kossoff, 1972). The only other evidence that the grievant actually took a drink was a statement to that effect made to his supervisor by the other employee involved in the incident. However, that evidence, too, was rejected as hearsay since the employee was not called to testify.

In *Comco Metal Products, Ltd.*, 58 LA 279, 280 (Brown, 1972), the arbitrator gave no weight to an accusation by a fellow employee that the two grievants had been drinking from and passing around a bottle of gin in the ladies' room since the employee, though apparently available to testify, was not called by the company. "In the nature of the allegations and the seriousness of the penalty imposed, this type of evidence cannot be accepted as truth that the offenses were committed as she alleged."

[107]For example, the arbitrator accepted a foreman's written report which was supported by a *second* supervisor's report that he found one full and one empty whiskey bottle in the place where the report stated the grievant had been pouring liquid from a bottle into a plastic container and drinking it. The grievance was denied. (*Chrysler Corp., Airtemp Div.*, 67–1 ARB ¶8135 (Kabaker, 1967).

my own eyes" type of evidence—to prove that an employee was drinking on the job.[108] Since most on-premises drinking takes place surreptitiously, suspicion often is aroused only by the discovery of a bottle or beer can or some other telltale sign.

> TWO CRITERIA:
>
> Circumstantial evidence is as strong proof of drinking as direct evidence, or even stronger, *when:*
>
> 1. The facts *point convincingly* to the conclusion that the employee must have been drinking (and cannot be accounted for by some other explanation); *and*
> 2. The facts themselves are solidly established. (Credibility plays a part here as it does in direct evidence cases, though more indirectly.)

The Two Criteria in Practice

SUPPOSE: *Too long at lunch*

Miles Foreman begins to think something might be wrong when Harry Workman and Mike Armstrong fail to show up on time after lunch. Recalling that he smelled alcohol on their breaths when they first reported in, he goes in search of them and finally spots them coming out of the No. 4 hacking station. He directs them to go back to work.

Checking the hacking station, Foreman finds seven full cans of beer—still cold—in a paper bag, and a number of empty cans on the floor. When he speaks with Workman and Armstrong shortly thereafter, he sees that Workman is having trouble speaking and his eyes are bloodshot.

So what did the facts add up to? According to the company, they pointed straightway to the conclusion that Workman and Armstrong were drinking, and the company forthwith fired both of them. Hold on, said the union; the grievants had drunk some beer before work that day—but that was all. Not so, said the arbitrator. Preshift drinking could not explain away the following facts:

[108]Arbitrator Shanker: "[T]he Union urges that drinking must be actually witnessed while it is taking place, or at least proven by direct evidence, such as medical tests given to prove that alcohol actually was in the system. . . . This argument is also rejected." (*Browning-Ferris Industries of Ohio, Inc.*, 77 LA 289, 292–93 (1981)).

• Testimony indicated that the smell of alcohol did not diminish in the course of their shift—as it would have if Workman and Armstrong had had a beer only before work, as they claimed:

• They were away from their work area for an extended period, even after having been told to return by Foreman;

• They were seen coming out of the hacking station where the cold cans of beer were found immediately after their exit;

• The hacking station was an unlighted and unheated area, and Workman and Armstrong had no good reason to be there;

• A photograph of the area showed a wet spot around a discarded beer can, which suggested very recent drinking;

• At least Workman showed physical signs of having been drinking.

Outcome: The conclusion that drinking had been going on draws more than ample support from the foregoing facts.[109]

In this case, since none of the facts was questioned by the union, the sole problem of proof was what those facts meant. The following case illustrates the part that credibility may play when a key fact is in dispute.

SUPPOSE: *One "empty"—then two*

Dave Powers enters the locker room one morning and spots an empty Budweiser beer can in a trash barrel. As he washes his hands, an unopened can in Harry Workman's open locker catches his eye. He picks up the can, finds that it is cold, replaces it and goes immediately to the Dispatch Office to call Workman's supervisor, Miles Foreman, to find out what the procedure is for questioning Workman.

Workman happens to be in the Dispatch Office and announces that he is going to wash his hands because his truck was dirty. Powers follows him back to the locker room and waits outside for about 15 minutes, during which time no one else enters or leaves. When Workman leaves he immediately goes in and finds a second empty beer can in the trash barrel along with the first. Workman's locker is now empty of beer.

The company concludes from Powers' story that the only explanation for the beer's disappearance was that Workman drank it while he was in the locker room. But not only does the union deny that Workman has been drinking; Workman swears that he had no beer in his locker. Why would he be so foolish as to leave his locker open if there was beer in it, plainly visible? And if Powers was telling the truth, why didn't he confront Workman when he was supposedly drinking the beer and catch him in the act?

[109] *Spartek, Inc.*, 77–1 ARB ¶8230 (Gibson, 1977).

So the case comes down in part to who was to be believed—Workman or Powers.

The outcome: Powers was credible; Workman was not. Workman damaged his credibility significantly at the hearing by not telling the truth about his prior disciplinary record, leading the arbitrator to doubt his truthfulness about the beer cans as well. And the fact that Powers failed to catch Workman red-handed did not in itself make his story untrue.[110] The events, as Powers reported them, could hardly be explained in any other way. Workman's discharge was therefore sustained.[111]

ASK YOURSELF:

When an employee is charged with drinking on the job on the basis of circumstantial evidence, the following factors should be considered (The more "Yes" answers, the better the case):

- Was an alcoholic beverage (or empty container) found in the employee's physical possession—in his hand, in his pocket—or in a location where it is reasonable to conclude that it belonged to him or was under his control, such as in his locker, lunch box, tool kit or immediate work area?

[110]The arbitrator pointed out, "Had [H.] [the manager] confronted [P.] [the grievant] with the can of beer in his locker, [P.] would have denied it was his—as he does. [H.'s] not going into the locker room does not make his story untrue. Perhaps a detective would have entered the locker room to try to catch [P.] drinking the beer, but [H.] is not trained in surveillance."

It should be noted, however, that another arbitrator might have taken the view that the manager was obligated to confront Workman about the beer in the locker as soon as he saw him in the dispatch office, rather than waiting for him to commit the further offense of drinking it.

[111]*Allegheny Ludlum Steel Corporation,* 66–2 ARB ¶8656 (Crawford, 1966). For other examples of "circumstantial evidence" cases, see *Walgreen Co.,* 66 LA 443, 446 (Larkin, 1976) ("The evidence of his having made an unscheduled stop at a tavern and leaving the tavern with a brown paper bag, later found in his truck with a partly consumed bottle of Scotch, was clear evidence of a dischargeable offense. Two of the three Company representatives who were observing the grievant's conduct testified that they smelled liquor on L—'s breath. . . ."); *Nevada Power Co.,* 77–1 ARB ¶8223, 3974 (McNaughton, 1977) ("Mr. [B.] did not see the grievant drink from the bottle. However, the odor of beer was strong. Mr. [B.] saw the grievant carrying a brown bottle with a Coors label, the grievant held it behind him when he saw Mr. [B.], he did not deny the accusation or prove that it was orange soda pop as he could easily have done at the time."); *Farm Stores, Inc.,* 83–2 ARB ¶8447 (Hanes, 1983) ("It is more than a suspicious circumstance that there was one can of beer on the driver's [J.'s] side of the box and one can of beer on the helper's [the grievant's] side of the box and that both cans of beer were partially consumed and the [J.] was drinking from both cans.")

Also take a look at *McCormick & Baxter Creosoting Co.,* and *Kaiser Sand and Gravel,* both KEY CASES IN DETAIL.

- If an empty can or container has been located, is it certain that it contained an alcoholic beverage?
- Is the evidence fresh—for example, is an empty beer can cold and/or moist, or is it dusty, as if it had been discarded some time previously?
- If the physical evidence was not found in the employee's work area, or in another place under his control, is there evidence that the grievant was in the area where the evidence was found?
- Did the employee show any physical signs of drinking, such as alcohol on his breath?
- Did the employee have the opportunity to drink?
- Were all avenues of investigation explored and no relevant evidence neglected?

Once a convincing "chain of circumstances" has been established, drinking will normally be accepted as proved *unless* the employee can offer some other credible explanation for the same facts.[112]

The grievant's story "washed"—just barely—for example, in *George A. Hormel & Co.*, 69 LA 853 (Lorimer, undated). A management official in that case caught the grievant placing a beer can in a file drawer. The can contained some beer; it had condensation on it as well as lip marks around the opening, and, according to the manager, the grievant had alcohol on his breath and bloodshot eyes. But the grievant claimed that he had found the can on his way into the plant and did not want to throw it into the trash can outside because he feared that would get other employees in trouble. He explained his bloodshot eyes by saying he had been up late the night before, had risen early, and had had a long drive to the plant.

The arbitrator had his doubts about the grievant's story, but he found it at least as plausible as the company's and therefore decided the company had not sustained its burden of proof.

For a case in which the arbitrator found the grievant's story too hard to swallow, see *Kaiser Sand & Gravel*, KEY CASES IN DETAIL, where two empty port wine bottles somehow made their way into the cab of the grievant's truck.

[112]Arbitrator Ipavec: "The conclusion which is deduced from circumstantial evidence is based on common sense and everyday observation. When such a deduction has been made from a chain of circumstances, the party in rebuttal must come forth with evidence which weakens the chain of circumstances." (*Diamond International*, 82–2 ARB ¶8326, 4471 (1982))

CAVEAT: A flask in the locker is not necessarily whiskey down the hatch.

Just as the fact that an employee has been drinking does not *necessarily* mean that he is under the influence, the fact that an employee is shown to be in possession of alcohol does not *in itself* amount to proof that he has been drinking.

Suggestive though it may be, simple "possession" cannot be elevated to "drinking" without additional evidence, direct or circumstantial, that the beer or the booze made its way from its container down the grievant's throat, as the case of *Anvan Industries, Inc.,* 72–2 ARB ¶8516 (Kossoff, 1972) illustrates. The grievant frankly admitted he had had a can of beer in his hand, but he said he intended to pour it out because he thought his friend who had been drinking from it had had enough. The arbitrator declined to credit hearsay testimony offered by the company that he had actually drunk from the can and reinstated him, since under the contract only drinking—not possession—could lead to summary discharge.

III. POSSESSION OF AN ALCOHOLIC BEVERAGE

As with drinking on company premises, possession of an alcoholic beverage may be proved by either direct or circumstantial evidence.

SUPPOSE: *"I saw it in his hand."*

When plant security receives an anonymous phone tip that a party is going on in the dispatcher's office, two security officers set out to investigate. Entering the office, Dick Sargent sees four employees, one of whom, Harry Workman, is holding a plastic glass containing whiskey. His partner, Bill Brass, sees Mike Armstrong place a whiskey bottle in the refrigerator. Workman and Armstrong later deny any connection with the liquor, claiming they didn't notice the bottle and glass until the guards picked them up.

The key issue was credibility. Sargent did not know Workman, and he had no reason to pinpoint Workman as the guilty party from among the four employees present. He had a clear, close, and unobstructed view, and was backed up by Brass, who, though his attention was focused on Armstrong, had Workman in his line of vision. Workman, on the other hand, failed at the scene of the party to deny that the glass was his, remaining silent even when Sargent asked him point blank, "It's yours, isn't it?"

The outcome: Sargent was more credible, and Workman was properly suspended for possession of alcohol.[113]

***SUPPOSE:** The logical explanation*

Miles Foreman and his leadman, Ed Leader, are standing on the outside loading dock discussing parking problems when they see Harry Workman arrive for his shift, over an hour late, and enter the plant carrying a brown paper bag containing something square. Suspicious, they follow. By the time they catch up with him, Workman is coming out of the coat room—minus the paper bag. In the room they find only a single paper bag; it is inside the refrigerator, and contains four cans of beer.

What's the explanation? According to the company, the beer must have been Workman's. Workman denies it, claiming that the bag he was observed carrying contained only old clothes. He fails to produce the clothes, however, so the company's conclusion is accepted by the arbitrator and Workman's suspension is upheld.[114]

Proof in "possession" cases, whether it hangs on direct *or* circumstantial evidence, often turns on one of the following three questions:

SUPPOSE NO. 1: Whose *was it?*

A security guard notices Harry Workman "bobbing" up and down near a car parked in the company lot. When he gets to the car, he finds Workman squatting down by a rear wheel. Near the rear wheel is a styrofoam cup containing liquid which proved to be wine. Workman denies that the cup belongs to him, explaining that he had stopped to remove some "slag" from his shoe on his way to move his car.

[113]*General Electric Co.*, 74 LA 25 (Spencer, 1979). Credibility likewise decided the case of *Jehl Cooperage Co.*, 75 LA 901 (Odom, 1980). The grievant denied that a supervisor had found him in a dressing room holding a half-empty gin bottle, but tripped himself up in a subsequent meeting when he asked the supervisor if he had actually seen him take a drink. To the arbitrator, that question betrayed the fact that the grievant *knew* the supervisor had not seen him drinking and "virtually admits his possession of the gin bottle."

[114]*Diamond International Corp.*, 82-2 ARB ¶8326 (Ipavec, 1982). In *Alcolac Chemical Corp.*, 55 LA 306 (Robertson, 1970), circumstantial evidence convincingly proved possession where the grievants drove a forklift off company premises; stopped at a liquor store; and shortly after they returned, were observed whispering together close to where a paper bag containing a half-pint of whiskey was subsequently found. Their explanation that they merely left the plant to "road test" the forklift was not believable.

The outcome: No bottle or flask was found on Workman's person or in the vicinity of his car; the guard did not smell alcohol on his breath. Thus the company failed to prove that the cup of wine belonged to Workman.[15]

SUPPOSE NO. 2: What *was it?*

Mary Foreman enters a room and sees Harry Workman pouring liquid from a bottle into a cup. She confiscates the bottle, but not the cup. The residue in the bottle is tested and found to contain alcohol. Workman swears the only thing in the cup was coffee—when he was caught by Foreman, he even offered to let her taste it!

The outcome: Because Foreman failed to get the "best" and most conclusive evidence available that Workman was in possession of alcohol—the cup—the arbitrator decided that the company had not satisfactorily proved its case.[116]

SUPPOSE NO. 3: *Can the possession be described as* innocent?

Harry Workman is observed in the parking lot by a security guard, Dick Sargent, holding a whiskey bottle. Workman, a black, has been promoted recently, resulting in some resentment by other employees. He explains to Sargent that his car has been vandalized during the past few days, and he has come out to the parking lot to check it during his break. He claims he found the bottle in the car and was in the process of throwing it away when Sargent spotted him.

[115]*Kast Metals Corp.*, 65 LA 783 (Davis, 1975). The arbitrator agreed that the grievant's actions were peculiar; but the company's case was stranger still:

"But why would any man, even the worst alcoholic, be found bobbing up and down presumably taking a drink, 15 minutes before his shift ended, and then squat by a cup which when discovered was still ½ to ¾ full. No one saw him in possession of the cup. No one smelled alcohol on his breath. No one observed that he was under the influence of alcohol. No one found a bottle or flask. No analysis was made of the contents of the cup. . . ."

[116]*Home Health Hospital of the Daughters of Jacob*, 74–1 ARB ¶8234 (Sandler, 1974). Another arbitrator might not have held the employer to such a stringent standard of proof; however, the case serves as "clear notice" to the supervisor about the kind of thoroughness in evidence-gathering which some arbitrators *may* expect.

In another case involving the "what," the Union contended that the Company had not proved that the liquid found in a jar in the grievant's lunch box was really wine, because the Company had not had the liquid tested. But the Arbitrator accepted the supervisors' identification of the liquid by its smell and taste. (*Pittsburgh Steel Co.*, 63–2 ARB ¶8756 (McDermott, 1963)).

The outcome: The arbitrator found Workman's story credible and ruled that he had been caught in "involuntary possession" of the whiskey.[117]

CHECKLIST—ASK YOURSELF:

The company normally has strong evidence of possession if it can answer "Yes" to the following questions:

- Is it securely established that the alcohol belonged to the employee charged with its possession?
- Has the beverage been positively identified as alcohol?
- Has the possibility that the employee was in possession of the alcohol "innocently" been ruled out?

Also take a look at the Checklists for Direct and Circumstantial Evidence of Drinking (pp. 89 and 103).

[117] *Holcroft Co.,* 55 LA 907 (Keefe, 1970). Also see cases cited in Chapter 2, REASONABLE RULES, p. 15. Wrongful intent was considered proved, however, in *Comco Metal Products, Ltd.,* 58 LA 279, 281 (Brown, 1972): "[H]ad an employee purchased a bottle during the lunch break, for instance, and brought it back to work to be taken home later . . . there would be no offense, but here the bottle was at least half empty and the circumstances . . . raised reasonable suspicions of wrongful intent. This, then, called for a reasonable explanation by F— and none was given."

Chapter 6

EQUAL TREATMENT

"Has the Employer applied its rules, orders and penalties even-handedly and without discrimination to all employees?"

INTRODUCTION

> *Arbitrator T. McDermott:* "Discrimination against an individual occurs when it is shown that there is unequal treatment of that employee as against others."[1]

Since the passage of the 1964 Civil Rights Act, the term "discrimination" as commonly used has come increasingly to refer to the unequal, or disparate, treatment of an individual by reason of that individual's race, sex, or less often, national origin or religion. Within the specific context of just cause, however, "discrimination" has broader implications. Just cause prohibits the unequal treatment of one employee, as compared with others, for *any* reason that is not directly related to his performance as an employee.

Just cause also contemplates that an employee cannot be disciplined for actions for which other employees have not been penalized. In alcohol cases, the Equal Treatment test most frequently causes problems when the company has been lax about enforcing its no-alcohol rules. If employees have previously broken the rules with impunity, *and* with supervisors' knowledge, a grievant who is "busted" for a drinking violation can complain with justification that he has been arbitrarily and capriciously singled out for unequal treatment, i.e., has been the victim of "discrimination."

Same principle, different "clothes." Claims of unequal treatment can also be made if some employees have been penalized less severely than others without some business-related basis (e.g., longer service or

[1] *Vulcan Mold & Iron Co.*, 70–1 ARB ¶8117, 3411 (1969).

a better work record), for the same type of violation. Lax rule enforcement and inconsistent administration of penalties both lead to the same result: disparate treatment of one employee, compared with others, and a failure by the company on the "Equal Treatment" test that is likely to cause an arbitrator to wipe out, or at least reduce, a disciplinary penalty even when the company has proved that misconduct was committed.

A PREVIEW

I. Lax or Inconsistent Enforcement of No-Alcohol Rules
- Rhymes and reasons
- Paying the piper: the results of lax enforcement
- "Cracking down," but with just cause
- The question of proof
  - The "should have known" question

II. Inconsistent Penalties
- What makes penalties inconsistent and what can "even them out" again
- Rehabilitation for the chronic alcoholic: "unequal treatment"?

I. LAX OR INCONSISTENT ENFORCEMENT OF NO-ALCOHOL RULES

Arbitrator Keltner: "If the rule is worth making, it is worth being enforced consistently."[2]

RHYMES AND REASONS

Something of a paradox. It may seem paradoxical that rules designed to keep alcohol out of the workplace are universally approved as being reasonable and necessary but, at the same time, are not always enforced with the consistency that might be expected in the case of a rule whose purpose is to ensure employees' safety as well as to promote efficient production.

[2]*Libby, McNeill & Libby*, 70 LA 1028, 1033 (Keltner, 1978).

Many different factors may contribute to a climate in which supervisors are less than diligent about "policing" employees' behavior on the job or marching them up to the front office when violations come to light. But one reason many supervisors look the other way when they see evidence of drinking (or, at most, just tell the employee "on the q.t." not to let it happen again, or to go home "sick") is their feeling that an individual can do a little drinking now and then and still be a valued employee.

Misconduct of a special sort. Alcohol violations differ in this respect from violations of many other work rules. Few supervisors would wink at an act of insubordination, for example, since a refusal to obey orders challenges the basic authority of management to run its business. Nor would most supervisors tend to overlook acts of theft, which show a clear and willful disregard for the company's interests.

Drinking, however, does not strike at the heart of the employer-employee relationship in quite the same way. An employee can sneak a drink, or show up after lunch just a little "high" because he didn't think that second beer would affect him, and still be someone who cares about doing a good job and whom the company would hate to lose. Moreover, a supervisor may detect alcohol on an employee's breath and decide not to make an issue of it because he believes that someone can do his job without being cold sober—perhaps because he has had that experience himself.

PAYING THE PIPER: THE RESULTS OF LAX ENFORCEMENT

If supervision has been lax, for whatever reason, about previously calling alcohol offenders on the carpet, the company is likely to have a hard time when it concludes that things have gotten out of hand and action must be taken in a particular case of misconduct.

SUPPOSE: *"Guilty—yes; discharge—no"*

Harry Workman was discharged when the company uncovered overwhelming circumstantial evidence that he had been drinking on the job. About 10 months earlier, three other employees had been caught drinking and suspended, and the company posted a notice informing employees that anyone caught drinking in the future would be fired. So far, so good.

There was just one problem: A management witness testified that although the company had had problems with employees drinking after the notice was posted, none of them had been disciplined. The witness also admitted that he had suspected Workman himself of being intoxicated on several earlier occasions, but had done nothing about it.

The result: Despite the posting of the notice, the fact that the company had made no effort to enforce the rule prior to Workman's discharge fatally compromised its right to get tough with Workman. Under the circumstances, discharge could not be justified—only the lesser penalty of a suspension could be imposed.[3]

A company's failure to enforce its no-alcohol rule, as illustrated by the foregoing case, actually deals a serious blow to not one but two of the just-cause tests.

First is Equal Treatment. Other employees got away with on-the-job drinking, even though management knew what was going on; Workman was penalized. Just the fact of such disparate treatment is enough in most cases to lead an arbitrator to reduce, or even rescind, the penalty no matter what the offense—possession of alcohol, drinking, even intoxication.

But in some cases the sudden singling out of one employee for discipline may act as an invitation for the union to argue that it could not have been drinking that galvanized the company into action (since it had never found such action necessary before), but—aha!—it must have been *some other reason,* unrelated to alcohol. If that other reason happens to be one that could place the company in a bad light—such as, for example, the grievant's race or union activities—the company may find itself fighting a defensive battle for which it never signed on—even if the allegations have no foundation in fact. Even charges that an employee was the victim of a supervisor's personal grudge can tarnish that supervisor's reputation for fair dealing and thereby detract from his effectiveness back at the workplace. And where morale is concerned, the *appearance* of unfairness can be as damaging as unfairness itself.

[3] *McCormick and Baxter Creosoting Co.,* KEY CASES IN DETAIL. See also *American Meat Packing Co.,* 79 LA 1327 (Malinowski, 1982) (company knew of other employees who were drinking and smoking marijuana during working hours; grievants, singled out unfairly for discharge, were reinstated with back pay); *Automotive Pattern Co.,* 69 LA 424, 77–2 ARB ¶8435 (Daniel, 1977) (other employees who drank on their lunch hours merely sent home); *Genest-Midwest, Inc.,* 67–2 ARB ¶8569 (Allman, 1967) (even if grievants had reported to work, others had been getting away with same offense).

The second just-cause test that lax rule enforcement calls into question is Notice.

When employees drink, *and* supervisors know they do, *and* employees know they know they do—*and* on top of that nothing is done about it—a reasonable expectation is created that the rules will be allowed to lie there sleeping in the books and will not be enforced. If an employee knows the infractions of others have been condoned, or if he has broken the rules himself without being penalized, he may be able to claim that he believed it was okay to come to work a little "happy" or to have an occasional "pick me up" in the rest room.[4] In effect, the company has established what might be called a *"general" practice of lax enforcement* upon which the employee has reason to rely.

What might be called *a "limited or special" practice of lax enforcement* arises through situations such as the following:

- *Holiday drinking.* A limited practice often comes into being with respect to drinking and partying around Christmas, New Year's, and other holidays, when some supervisors are more likely to turn a blind eye—or even themselves to join in the festivities—than at other times of the year. The fact that it was holiday time in itself does not excuse an alcohol rule violation; but discipline may not hold up if management has *condoned* holiday drinking in the past even if the rules are strictly enforced as a general matter.[5]
- *Past practice and the single supervisor.* By no means does the entire management staff have to look the other way when alcohol rules

[4]In addition to *McCormick & Baxter Creosoting Co.,* KEY CASES IN DETAIL, see *Bi-State Development Agency,* 74–2 ARB ¶8687 (Mikrut, 1974), where the arbitrator overturned the discharge of a bus driver who reported for work under the influence, despite the safety hazards involved in his job, because six months earlier the employer had allowed him to go on working when he was in a similar condition.

[5]"[W]ith regard to the celebration of the last day before the Christmas holiday, there is no dispute between the parties that, for many years, this had been a day of gay abandon on the part of management and employees alike. Hence, despite the existence of the formal rule against drinking on the premises, I would have been constrained to rule that past practice created a situation in which the Company was estopped from enforcing the prohibition, as to conduct on that particular day." So the arbitrator found in *American Trailers, Inc.,* 73–2 ARB ¶8348, 4281–82 (Merrill, 1973). He upheld the grievant's suspensions only because the company had given notice that it intended to tighten enforcement of the rule shortly before the holiday on which they were caught drinking. In *Wagner Electric Corp.,* 57 LA 10 (Erbs, 1971), where no such notice had been given, previous supervisorial slackness about holiday drinking led the arbitrator to convert the grievant's discharge for drinking to a suspension without back pay.

are violated for a past practice to come into being. When a single supervisor acquiesces in any kind of drinking, limited or otherwise, he may lead employees to believe they can safely continue to violate a rule against such misconduct.

SUPPOSE: *"Sauce for the goose"*

During his lunch, Harry Workman meets a friend who used to work in his department. His friend has just become a father and gives Workman a bottle of bourbon to take back to work with him so that his old friends can celebrate "on him." Workman returns to work, sets up an impromptu "bar," and a little party begins. When management finds out, Workman is fired (though his discharge is later commuted to a 30-day suspension) and five other employees are suspended as well.

The catch: Miles Foreman, the immediate supervisor of all six employees, had brought in a bottle one or two months previously to celebrate his daughter's marriage.

The outcome: Reduced suspensions for all five employees who availed themselves of their old friend's "hospitality." "There is no doubt in the mind of the arbitrator that these five employees felt that a drink on company property, under the circumstances related here, would not have resulted in the punishment which they received. . . .

"If the rule would have been strictly enforced and not glossed over by persons in authority whenever it was to their convenience to do so, different results would have been obtained."[6]

• *Drinking off premises.* When management is permissive about off-premises drinking during lunch breaks or before a shift, employees may get the idea that the company is not serious about preventing employees from coming to work after having downed a couple. They may even believe it is also quite all right to "have a shot" on company premises. One arbitrator, for example, was not impressed with testimony that a company was waging "a vigorous campaign against the ravages of intoxication" when management personnel were buying drinks for employees at lunch:

[6]*Labor Standards Ass'n, Gimbel Brothers,* 61–3 ARB ¶8899 (Di Leone, 1961).

See also *Luck Mining Co.,* 69–1 ARB ¶8050 (Hayes, 1968): "Drinking on the job since February 15, 1968 by employees with the consent, approval and participation of the Foreman is an undisputed fact. Notwithstanding the fact that the Foreman was guilty of the most wrongful violation of his duty and responsibility as a Company supervisor, the Company is bound by his conduct in supervising Grievant and the other employees involved."

"There appears to be some incompatibility between an anti-drinking campaign and management encouragement of drinking at a bar during lunch. This is not to suggest that such practice increases intoxication. On the other hand, it assuredly does not enhance sobriety."[7]

The key question in all these cases is *what can employees reasonably expect?* If the company's enforcement of no-alcohol rules has been lax or spotty, or even downright permissive, it cannot change those "rules" at will—at least not without notice.

CRACKING DOWN—BUT WITH JUST CAUSE

The fact that a company has been haphazard about rule enforcement in the past does not mean that it cannot decide that enough is enough at some point and crack down.

"The Company has the right to take steps to tighten discipline, but its agreement with the Union, and general labor relations principles, require that when the Company has tolerated a condition and decides to end its toleration, *there must be some indication of the change in policy.*"[8]

The Equal Treatment test requires that the company not give "indication of a change in the policy" by suddenly swooping down on the first offender who comes to its attention, even though making an example of someone might succeed in bringing the company's warning message home to other employees. The company can, however, put employees on notice *in advance*—before anyone at all is disciplined—that in the future any violation of the "no alcohol" rule will result in discipline. In order to make it unmistakably clear that, no matter what may have gone on in the past, the company means business about

[7]*Freightliner Corp.;* KEY CASES IN DETAIL. Although supervisors were not directly involved, the fact that management condoned lunch-hour drinking contributed to the arbitrator's decision that discharge was too harsh in *Southern Indiana Gas Co.,* 71–1 ARB ¶8226 (Edelman, 1971), since the small amount of beer which the grievant drank on working time was no more than other employees frequently drank—with the company's knowledge—at lunch.

[8]*Genest-Midwest, Inc.,* 67–2 ARB ¶8569, 4994 (Allman, 1967). Another statement of the same principle: "From the evidence I find that this problem, per se, was not new to this Company. In view of the problem in the old facility it seems only logical that reposting and stressing the rule should have been done at both the old and new facilities as it is patent that no adequate control program existed at the old plant." (*Industrial Plastics Corp.,* 58 LA 546, 548 (Willingham, 1972))

changing its practices and that henceforth the old rule will be given new teeth, such notice should go beyond merely reposting or restating the old rule.

TAKE A LOOK AT the following notice in which employees were informed in no uncertain terms how a crackdown on a persistent holiday drinking problem might proceed:

"NOTICE"

> "As we approach the Holiday Season, we would like to remind you that drinking and work do not mix. Last year we had some bad experiences here at the plant with people reporting for work under the influence of alcohol."
>
> "You are reminded that this is a violation of the Shop Rules and cannot be tolerated. Therefore, you are asked not to report for work under the influence of alcohol. Also, there will be no alcoholic beverages admitted into the plant at all. Violations will result in severe disciplinary action."[9]

Such a notice may be posted on appropriate bulletin boards; sent to the union; duplicated and distributed to employees individually; communicated orally by supervisors where feasible—whatever method or combination of methods will get the message across.

Thereafter, of course, the company has to stick to its guns. Management can announce changes in policy until the cows come home—but (as in the "SUPPOSE" on page 118) if people start drinking again and if no one is disciplined, the company is right back where it started, done in by the principle that notice is a matter not only of what management *says* but of what it *does*.

On the other side of the coin, if the company has indeed undertaken an energetic and sustained program to curb alcohol violations,

[9]*Burnham Corp.*, 73–1 ARB ¶8036, 3144 (Pollock, 1973). Tightening of enforcement was communicated to employees at another company by means of this notice: "Lately we have had employees either reporting to work under the influence of alcohol or drugs or becoming under the influence after the shift has started. The work rules call for the first offense being a Three Day Disciplinary Lay Off, with the next offense being Discharge. I cannot think of many quicker ways of getting injured than to attempt to work after drinking alcohol or taking drugs. Please have respect for yourself, your family and your fellow employees and don't drink until you get off work. For your safety and the safety of others around you, this rule will be enforced." (*Hayes-Albion Corp.*, 76 LA 1005, 1006–1007 (Kahn, 1981))

most arbitrators would be reluctant to dilute the company's efforts by reducing disciplinary penalties even in cases which otherwise might call for a different approach.[10]

THE QUESTION OF PROOF

The union has obligations, too. For the union to get discipline set aside on the basis of a defense of lax enforcement, it needs more than unsupported claims that the company has let people get away scot free with violations of the rule. The union must *prove,* with convincing testimony, that *specific violations have taken place* and that *management was definitely aware that such events had been taking place*—the more names, dates, and places the better. Thus, testimony in one case that the grievant's heavy drinking habits were "common knowledge" in the plant was of no help to his defense, where union witnesses could cite no specific occasions on which he had been drinking on company premises in a supervisor's presence.[11]

Moreover, condoned conduct must have been *relatively recent*—stale practices will not carry much weight—and must be *similar in nature* to the offense which the grievant committed.

EXAMPLE NO. 1: *Long ago and far away*

> The union presented unassailable evidence that employees who worked oven jobs had made a practice of taking brandy and tea in lieu of salt tablets for the heat. The evidence was given barely a nod by the arbitrator; the union was merely grasping at straws because the practice had lapsed some 20 years earlier.[12]

[10]That was the case, for example, in *AMF Lawn & Garden Div.*, 64 LA 988 (Wyman, 1975). Faced with a serious alcohol problem, the company had employed a security force, undertaken lunch box and parcel inspections, and reemphasized its rules against alcohol use on Company premises. Said the arbitrator: "Standing alone as an isolated case, discharge for the first offense of the sole act of possessing alcoholic beverages on Company premises (as opposed to consumption, which this case involves additionally) must be adjudged as too severe. But the act . . . exists in a web of circumstances contained in a calculated, publicized, company-initiated program designed to solve a problem of some magnitude." The grievant's discharge was upheld.

[11]*Liberty Baking Co.*, 64–1 ARB ¶8226 (Kreimer, 1964). See also *Northwest Airlines, Inc.*, 1975 ARB ¶8207, 3871 (Turkus, 1975): "The affirmative defenses that NWA has condoned or waived the enforcement of the 24–hour rule in its application as to others similarly situated and that the grievant was the victim of disparate treatment are utterly without substance and merit. Not a single situation has been demonstrated that NWA has knowingly failed to discharge any cockpit crew member for a violation of the 24–hour rule or that there has been disparate punishment in this case."

[12]*Liberty Baking Co.*, Note 11 above.

EXAMPLE NO. 2: Before the crackdown

An incident in which the grievant had a drink with his foreman when work was interrupted during a snowstorm was found not to bind the company because the incident took place before the company announced a "crackdown" on drinking and began enforcing that policy consistently by means of the discharge penalty. The grievant's discharge was therefore upheld.[13]

EXAMPLE NO. 3: No comparison

"While testimony from Union witnesses indicates that some degree of drinking occurred in earlier years [on the last workday before Christmas], the union failed to show that these earlier affairs had the organization, supplies, or verve of the 1979 gala"—an openly conducted, drunken "free for all". Nothing in the past practice could reasonably have led employees to believe that misconduct of those dimensions would likewise be condoned. Discipline was therefore upheld.[14]

The "Should Have Known" Question

SUPPOSE the following testimony on cross-examination by the company's general foreman:

"Q. There have been a lot of bottles in the plant, regularly?"
"A. There have been, but I haven't seen any recently. There've been bottles gathered up for some time—I'll admit that—but I don't think drinking has been a regular thing. It comes and goes, unless steps are taken to prevent it."

And then testimony by the foreman:

"Q. Drinking has gone on repeatedly in the plant by other employees?"
"A. There has been some drinking."

Finally, the assistant foreman (being asked about his testimony that the janitor had found four empty vodka bottles on the day of the grievant's discharge):

"Q. It isn't unusual for the janitor to sweep up bottles in the plant?"
"A. Not really. I have seen this occur several times."

[13]*Derse Advertising Co.*, 69–2 ARB ¶8474 (Sembower, 1969). Past history was also effectively wiped out by an announced tightening of the rules in *American Trailers, Inc.*, 73–2 ARB ¶8348 (Merrill, 1973); and *Prescolite*, 71 LA 613 (Bridgewater, 1978).

[14]*Anaconda Co., New Mexico Operations*, 80–2 ARB ¶8380 (Cohen, 1980).

No one stated that any supervisor had ever caught an employee in the act of drinking; no one spoke of employees walking around reeking of booze.

Does this make for lax enforcement? You bet, said the arbitrator. He agreed with the union that:

> "[T]he rule against drinking had not, prior to [the grievant's] termination, been enforced with that degree of effectiveness and consistency which might fairly have been regarded as a clear indication to Grievant or any other employee, that one more drinking episode would warrant discharge.
>
> . . . IN VIEW OF THE DEGREE OF LAXITY WHICH HAD PREVAILED IN THE ENFORCEMENT OF RULE 9 . . . the doctrine of just cause contemplates that, UNDER SUCH CIRCUMSTANCES, the Grievant here should have been issued a clear-cut warning to the effect that another violation of Rule 9 would mean his discharge."[15]

This conclusion stands for the proposition that there are some circumstances in which management may be charged with having a kind of "constructive knowledge" that employees are breaking the rules and getting away with it. To put it another way, management *should have known* what was going on, and can therefore be held responsible for not putting a stop to a practice just as surely as if employees had been caught red-handed without being penalized.

In part, the "should have known" principle is a matter of Notice again. If empty vodka bottles are regularly left around where anyone might find them, and no one from management comes sniffing around the break areas or makes any visible effort to find out where they are actually coming from, employees may get the idea (perhaps not intended) that the company is not overly concerned about alcohol violations.

The Investigation test also comes into play.

[15] *Ward Furniture Mfg. Co.*, 63–2 ARB ¶8826, 5663 (Boles, 1963). To the same effect, Arbitrator Keltner in *Libby, McNeill & Libby*, 70 LA 1029, 1032–33 (1978): "If the Company disciplines only those employees it apprehends and does not make concerted and serious effort to spread its surveillance equally and evenly throughout the plant, it is *not* fulfilling the standard procedure of evenhanded application. Application of a rule must involve the efforts to provide surveillance as well as the treatment of those employees caught in violation."

> THE CONNECTION—In re: "Investigation"
>
> The Investigation test requires the company to inquire thoroughly into the facts *after* a violator has been caught and discipline is contemplated.
>
> Additionally, that test may be interpreted to require the company as a preventive measure to make positive efforts to identify violators and to monitor employees' activities more closely when it is given reason to believe that the rules are being flouted.

Does the "should have known" test go too far? A manager might very well begin to wonder at this point—"Supervisors aren't policemen," he can be imagined protesting. "People tend to drink on the sly, you know, and supervisors can't spend all their time poking their noses into people's thermos bottles trying to catch them breaking the rules. After all, employees know what the rules say. Just because we can't be everywhere at once doesn't mean we shouldn't have the right to fire somebody when we finally do catch him in the act."

He has a point. Obviously, *it's a matter of degree.* Where violations, even if fairly widespread, have been well concealed, the company cannot be faulted for not instructing all its supervisors to drop everything to play Dick Tracy. There are also situations that are extremely difficult to police even if the employer tried to do so—such as in the case of off-premises drinking by truck drivers and other employees who work in the field.[16]

But where the union can show that the company has found obvious and repeated evidence of alcohol violations, and tried neither to identify the culprits nor to prevent further misconduct—whether by means of crackdown notices, routine lunchbox searches, or observation of likely drinking locations—the burden would then normally shift to the company to show why its inactivity should not be considered lax enforcement and condonation.

[16]A rule prohibiting airline employees from consuming any alcohol within 24 hours before reporting for duty was found by one arbitrator to be "difficult, if not impossible, to police and enforce," and for that reason even evidence that there had been "wholesale violations" of the rule did not establish acquiescence on the company's part. *Northwest Airlines, Inc.*, 56 LA 837, 842 (Wyckoff, 1971).

II. INCONSISTENT PENALTIES

WHAT MAKES PENALTIES INCONSISTENT—AND WHAT CAN "EVEN THEM OUT"?

Unequal treatment wears a somewhat different set of clothes when the company, though conscientious about enforcing its alcohol rules and disciplining the violators, arbitrarily hands out different penalties for comparable offenses.

> *Arbitrator Rose:* "There were three day suspensions, demotions, warning letters, shift changes. And these lesser penalties occurred sometimes for repeat offenders. . . . And it appears that the expectation among line management personnel in the instant matter was that the grievant would receive little, if any, discipline.
>
> "The paint foreman testified that the line manager informed him that the grievant was 'sent home to sober up' and would return the following morning. The personnel manager testified rather vaguely that he has terminated employees for being under the influence, and has not terminated others. . . .
>
> "The Arbitrator is not suggesting that penalties need be precisely identical, *but a pattern of consistency should be readily discernible.*" (Emphasis added.) (*Freightliner Corp.*, KEY CASES IN DETAIL)

SUPPOSE: *No second or third (or fourth) chance*

> Harry Workman is discharged for showing up at work intoxicated for the second time. However, some foremen have given other employees not only second but third (and sometimes fourth) "chances" for reporting to work in that condition before imposing discipline.
>
> *The outcome:* The Arbitrator found that disciplinary policy had been applied evenhandedly at the middle-management level, but first-line supervisors exercised considerable discretion, producing inconsistent penalties for the same offense. Discharge was reduced to a two-month suspension.[17]

If an employer imposes a more severe penalty on the grievant than that which other employees have received for the same type of misconduct, that penalty is likely to be reduced by an arbitrator *unless* some factor is present that justifies more severe treatment.

[17]*Aerojet Liquid Rocket Co.*, 75 LA 255 (Wollett, 1980).

FIVE CASES IN POINT:

CASE NO. 1:

Harry Workman and Mike Armstrong are both guilty of becoming intoxicated at lunch and reporting to work in that condition. Workman is discharged, while Armstrong receives only a one-week suspension and a warning—"unequal treatment" that the arbitrator upheld. Why?

Different work records. Workman had been previously warned in connection with an earlier drinking incident, while Armstrong's record was unblemished. "So it cannot be said that there was discrimination in the disciplinary action meted out."[18]

CASE NO. 2:

Harry Workman not only shows up for work intoxicated but compounds his misconduct by using abusive language to supervision and refusing to leave the premises. Although the company had not discharged other employees who reported under the influence, but merely sent them home, Workman's discharge is sustained.

The reason: aggravated misconduct. None of the employees who were dealt with more liberally had engaged in any additional offenses.[19]

CASE NO. 3:

Workman brings a bottle of bourbon onto company premises, sets up a temporary "bar," and provides ice, glasses, and mixer for himself and other employees. All are suspended for 30 days; however, the arbitrator reduces that penalty for all but Workman, who instigated the drinking party.

The deciding factor: greater responsibility. "If the principal wrongdoer . . . was given a one month disciplinary layoff, it cannot be equitable to apply the same penalty to the five grievants who committed a lesser offense."[20]

[18]*Ocean Spray Cranberries, Inc.*, 68–1 ARB ¶8252, 3880 (Sembower, 1969). Similarly, in *Spartek, Inc., Wall Tile Div.*, 77–1 ARB ¶8230 (Gibson, 1977), the discharge of one of two employees who were drinking on the job was sustained despite the fact that the other received a 2½-day suspension, since the first employee had relatively short service (about one year, as opposed to six years for the other) and had received four warnings during that time (for drinking before reporting to work, wandering from his work area, and absenteeism).

[19]*White Pine Copper Co.*, 63–2 ARB ¶8548 (Larkin, 1963). See also *Libby, McNeill & Libby*, 40 LA 717 (Davis, 1963).

[20]*Labor Standards Ass'n, Gimbel Brothers*, 61–3 ARB ¶8899 (Di Leone, 1961). The same principle was applied to the opposite effect in *Brown and Williamson Tobacco Corp.*, 52 LA 405, 69–2 ARB ¶8478, 4626 (Stouffer, 1969). Although he took a "hard line" view that discharge normally would not be too harsh a penalty, even for a first offense of drinking on the job, the arbitrator rescinded the grievant's discharge because the two real instigators, the employee who brought in the whiskey and the employee who made it available to the grievant, escaped without penalty; he commented that "the incident most likely would not have occurred but for [B.'s] misconduct. The temptation to violate the plant rule was placed before the grievant by this so-called friend."

CASE NO. 4:

The discharge of Harry Workman for bringing a bottle of gin onto company property is upheld, even though employees in the shipping and receiving department have received lesser penalties for alcohol violations.

What's different about Workman's case? Greater job hazards. Workman worked as a punch operator, a job which is described as "one of the most dangerous in the industry. . . . Suffice it to say that the Company has a responsibility to see that employees who have been drinking do not operate machines."[21]

CASE NO. 5:

In a case with a slightly different twist, the company attempted to justify the discharge of Helen Workman for the relatively "light" offense of bringing a bottle of whiskey into the plant by pointing out that it had discharged another employee previously for the same violation without protest from the union. But the arbitrator found one crucial factor that made the other employee's offense more serious.

Guilty intentions. Workman had forgotten the whiskey was in her purse and brought it into the plant unknowingly; the other employee had been well aware of what he was doing. Workman was reinstated with just a suspension.[22]

One factor that does not as a rule justify unequal penalties is degree of intoxication. As discussed in the chapter on proof, the gradations recognized in everyday life, from "high" or "happy" to "drunk" and on up to "dead drunk," "bombed," or "smashed," have no relevance at the workplace.

Arbitrator Geissinger: "If being under the influence of liquor or alcoholic beverage in any degree is just cause for mandatory discharge the Company is obligated by its own rule to discharge everyone found to be 'under the influence.' . . . The drunker of the two employees is in

[21]*Jehl Cooperage Co.*, 75 LA 901 (Odom, 1980). Most arbitrators would agree—but not all. In *Prescolite*, 71 LA 613, 619 (Bridgewater, 1978), the arbitrator refused to accept the grievant's job as a forklift driver as justification for his discharge on intoxication charges where an intoxicated employee who performed less hazardous work was merely sent home. Not to reinstate him, she found, "would unfairly discriminate against him solely on the basis of the job he held. . . ."

[22]*Packaging Corp. of America*, 56 LA 856 (Anrod, 1971).

> no greater violation than the one who is less drunk but still 'under the influence.' . . . If H— was not to be discharged, although admittedly 'under the influence,' C— should not have been discharged.[23]

Unequal penalties were also rejected where only the employees who admitted drinking at an impromptu party were disciplined while others who the company knew had also been drinking (but who did not admit it) were let off without penalty.[24] Another example: Mike Armstrong admitted that he had been drinking and said that Harry Workman, the grievant, was drinking with him. Workman's discharge was set aside because Armstrong got off with only a warning for his cooperation.[25]

Rehabilitation for the Chronic Alcoholic: "Unequal Treatment"?

Two kettles of fish

Employers have sometimes expressed concern that if an employee who suffers from chronic alcoholism is given the opportunity to rehabilitate himself instead of having to face the music (see Chapter 7, p. 145), a precedent may be set that could allow a nonalcoholic employee to protest his discharge or other penalty on "unequal treatment" grounds. Arbitrators have consistently held, however, that by taking a nondisciplinary approach to chronic alcoholics, the company does not waive its right to penalize employees whose use of alcohol is not a matter of illness but is within their control.[26]

[23]*Page Aircraft Mfg. Co.*, 56 LA 860, 862–63 (1971). In a case where 30 employees were given 30–day suspension for drinking at a Christmas party, the arbitrator refused to sustain the discharges of two of their fellow party-goers, who were dealt with more severely because they passed out. "All participated in an unauthorized activity on Company property where alcoholic beverages were consumed; all refused direct orders to return to work, in complete disregard of supervisory authority; and all were intoxicated on Company property. The fact that the Grievants had to be assisted out of the mine while the others walked out—but not in a straight line—seems to me to be a thin distinction for justifying such extremity in discipline." The grievants, too, were given 30–day suspensions. (*Anaconda Co.*, 80–2 ARB ¶8380 (Cohen, 1980).

[24]*Labor Standards Ass'n, Gimbel Brothers*, 61–3 ARB ¶8899 (Di Leone, 1961).

[25]*Browning-Ferris Industries of Ohio, Inc.*, 77 LA 289 (Shanker, 1981).

[26] See, e.g., *Armstrong Rubber Co.*, 77 LA 775 (Koven, 1981); *Golden Operations, CWC Castings Div. of Textron, Inc.*, 80–2 ARB ¶8543 (Ipavec, 1980). The same point is addressed in *Allied Employers, Inc.*, 79–1 ARB ¶8121 (Abernathy, 1978), where the arbitrator rejected as groundless the company's concern that if alcoholism were to be treated as an illness, for which an employee would be entitled to sick leave and other benefits, it would be unable to discharge employees for drinking or drunkenness on the job.

The more problematical issue

Sometimes equality of treatment among chronic alcoholics itself becomes an issue. Whatever special rehabilitation opportunities the company has afforded some chronic alcoholics in lieu of discipline, it must normally make available on the same basis to all other alcoholic employees. For example, where the grievant was not given the benefit of a company policy under which other employees were permitted to attend a rehabilitation clinic and be reemployed upon successful completion of the clinic's program, the arbitrator found that:

> "[I]t seems only fair that management in realizing that alcoholism had affected the attendance problems of its senior employees to a considerable degree in 1981, . . . should have been consistent in imposing its penalties to all on an equal basis. . . . In other words, grievant K— should have been offered the same privilege as others in the same boat, and the company by failing to apply its disciplinary policies in an even-handed manner can be said to be guilty of discriminating against this particular employee."[27]

The arbitrator went on to say that the company had the option of changing its policy if it wished to do so—but not without advance notice of any change.

[27]*Indianapolis Rubber Co.*, 79 LA 529, 534 (T. Gibson, 1982). Also see *Armstrong Rubber Co.*, Note 26 above.

Chapter 7

PENALTY

"Was the degree of discipline administered by the Employer in a particular case reasonably related to (a) the seriousness of the employee's *proven* offense, and (b) the record of the employee in his service with the employer?"

INTRODUCTION

Arbitrator Platt: "The inquiry must be not only whether the disciplined employee was guilty of the acts charged but also whether they were committed in the course of his employment and whether they constitute industrial misconduct. And, too, the inquiry must be into whether the penalty imposed is such a one as would appeal to fair minded persons, mindful of the customs of industrial life and of the standards of justice prevalent in the community."[1]

The question of penalty is one on which employers and unions have locked horns repeatedly, management often taking the position that, if misconduct has been proved, management and management alone should determine the proper penalty. An arbitrator, according to this view, has no business "substituting his judgment for that of management" (as the standard phrase goes), and may not reduce whatever discipline the employer has imposed on the grievant. Needless to say, unions reject that limited assessment of the arbitrator's authority under the just-cause standard.

The great majority of arbitrators also take the view that managerial judgments about penalty are fair game for arbitral inquiry where just cause is in issue. Using criteria like seriousness of the offense and the employee's past record, they have routinely reviewed the degree of

[1]*Republic Steel Corp.*, 23 LA 808 (1955).

discipline imposed in cases of alcohol-related offenses as well as other types of misconduct, in accordance with Arbitrator Daugherty's seventh and last just-cause test.[2]

A PREVIEW

I. What Makes a Penalty Proper?
- Up and down the scale of misconduct
  - Intoxication: the most serious offense
  - Drinking on the job: a lesser form of misconduct?
  - Possession of alcoholic beverages: the other end of the scale
  - To sum up
- Other penalty factors
  - Notice and practice—a dynamic duo
  - Presence (or absence) of additional misconduct
  - Safety factors
  - Past record and length of service

II. The Chronic Alcoholic

III. The Arbitrator and the Penalty
- What if one or more of the seven tests have not been satisfied?
- Three flavors in the creamery
- "What, then, shall the remedy be"?

I. WHAT MAKES A PENALTY PROPER?

Any discussion of what degree of discipline is proper for a particular act of misconduct starts out by considering the seriousness of the offense.

[2]The most frequently quoted statement of the "opposition view," that penalties decided upon by management normally should not be disturbed, is that of Arbitrator McCoy in *Stockham Pipe Fitting Co.,* 1 LA 160, 162 (1945): "The mere fact that management has imposed a somewhat different penalty or a somewhat more severe penalty than the arbitrator would have, if he had had the decision to make originally, is no justification for changing it. The minds of equally reasonable men differ." But McCoy goes on to say: "The only circumstance under which a penalty imposed by management can be rightfully set aside by an arbitrator are those where discrimination, unfairness, or capricious and arbitrary action are proved—in other words, where there has been abuse of discretion." Thus even he gives the arbitrator some room to maneuver.

> *Arbitrator McCoy:* "Offenses are of two general classes: (1) those extremely serious offenses such as stealing, striking a foreman, persistent refusal to obey a legitimate order, etc., which usually justify *summary discharge* without the necessity of prior warnings or attempts at corrective discipline; (2) those *less serious infractions* of plant rules or of proper conduct such as tardiness, absence without permission, careless workmanship, insolence, etc., which call not for discharge for the first offense (and usually not even for the second or third offense) but for *some milder penalty aimed at correction.*"[3]

Into which of these two categories do alcohol-related offenses fall? Are alcohol violations (in the words used by another arbitrator to describe the kinds of offenses that deserve summary discharge) "misconduct which has shown such a weakness of character in the employee that it would be improper to require the employer to assume the risks involved in continuing the offender in his employ"?[4] Or do they fall short of that extreme seriousness?

The answer depends initially on which type of misconduct is involved: intoxication, drinking, or possession of alcohol.

UP AND DOWN THE SCALE OF MISCONDUCT

Intoxication: The Most Serious Offense

Obviously the employee who is proved to be (or who admits being) under the influence of alcohol while on the job invites severe discipline. But does this most serious form of alcohol-related misconduct always (or almost always) justify discharge? Some arbitrators think it does.

> *Arbitrator Goetz:* "It goes without saying that drunkenness on the job is one of the most serious offenses of which an employee can be found guilty. As illustrated by the facts of this case, such misconduct represents a serious safety hazard to the individual involved and to his fellow employees—not to mention the interference with production and disruption of order in the Plant. Consequently, many arbitrators have held that such misconduct falls in the category of offenses for which *discharge is warranted without resort to prior corrective discipline.*"[5]

But a respectable number of arbitrators have also held that despite the seriousness of the offense, discharge for intoxication is not always called for; *"it depends,"* they say.

[3] *Huntington Chair Corp.*, 24 LA 490, 491 (1955).

[4] *McInerney Spring & Wire Co.*, 21 LA 80, 84 (1953).

[5] *Perk Foods Co.*, 78–1 ARB ¶8083, 3391 (1977) (emphasis added).

Arbitrator Koven: "For a first offense of drinking or intoxication, where the employee has a long and discipline-free (or relatively discipline-free) work record, and where no other special factors are present, many arbitrators have held that discharge is too severe a penalty and that instead, *some form of corrective discipline is called for* to put the grievant on clear notice that insobriety will not be tolerated at the workplace and to give him the opportunity to change his ways."[6]

Reporting to work intoxicated v. getting drunk at work: Are they equally serious for purposes of penalty?

TWO SCHOOLS OF THOUGHT:

(1) *Two different things,* says one group of arbitrators.

Arbitrator R. Smith: "[I]t is more serious to drink and become intoxicated on the job than to appear at work in an inebriated state. The employee who appears for work 'under the influence' can be turned away at the gate, before he actually attempts to start work."[7]

(2) *No distinction should be made,* say others.

Their reasoning? The employee who shows up for work under the influence is no more able to perform his work than the employee who gets drunk on the job. Besides, there is always a danger that an employee who comes to work drunk will not be spotted before he clocks in and begins work, so possible discharge is necessary as a deterrent to prevent that from happening.[8]

[6]*Armstrong Rubber Co.,* 77 LA 775 (1981).

[7]*McInerney Spring and Wire Co.,* 21 LA 80 (1953). See also *Land O' Lakes Bridgeman Creamery,* 65 LA 803 (Smythe, 1975); and *Koppers Co., Inc.,* 65–1 ARB ¶8013 (Loucks, 1964), where the arbitrator found that a company rule making reporting to work under the influence "subject to immediate discharge" was itself subject to a "reasonable application" test. Because the offense of reporting under the influence is more a matter of an employee's not meeting his obligation to keep himself fit for his employment than of putting people and property in danger, a first offense would call for being sent home with a warning; a second, however, would warrant discharge.

[8]*Safeway Steel Scaffolds of Georgia,* 34 LA 14 (Bonebrake, 1959). The "inability to work" consideration served to do in even a grievant who called his supervisor in advance to say that he had had too many drinks to perform his job, where the contract made coming on duty under the influence sufficent cause for discharge, and the grievant had had serious problems with absenteeism. (*Wells Badger Industries, Inc.,* 76 2 ARB ¶8435, 67 LA 56, (J. Jones, 1976)) But in another case, where the grievant had a "clean" 15–year record, the fact that he frankly disclosed to his foreman as soon as he arrived at the plant that he had been drinking and might be "borderline" on a sobriety test, his candor worked in his favor. The company itself reduced intended discharge to a written reprimand, which was endorsed as an appropriate penalty by the arbitrator.

Drinking on the Job: A Lesser Form of Misconduct?

Common sense might suggest that drinking that stops short of an employee's being under the influence is less grave an offense than intoxication, and would therefore, as a general rule, merit a milder penalty. Many arbitrators have agreed with that proposition.

> *Arbitrator Volz:* "A review of the arbitration cases discloses that the mere possession of a can of beer in a lunch bucket and a consumption on the premises do not warrant a discharge unless extremely aggravating circumstances are present."[9]

But other arbitrators have taken a strict view of drinking which recognizes little or no difference between being intoxicated and drinking on the job, pointing out that "drinking" may turn the corner into "drunk" in the twinkling of an eye (though it does not do so inevitably) and that the employer should have the right to take action *before* serious harm is done.

> *Arbitrator Updegraff:* "As is commonly known, 'drinking' leads to 'intoxication' and the latter leads to carelessness and other well-known difficulties and complications. . . . A few drinks may, for a considerable period, have little effect apparent to either the consumer or to others, then suddenly and without warning render the user helpless or apparently direct him to illogical, unpredictable, and greatly harmful movements. "The risks of such possibilities should not be upon either the employer or upon the fellow employees of the drinker."[10]

The logical conclusion of many arbitrators in the Updegraff camp: Discharge even for a first offense of "drinking only" is proper.

[9] *Altamil Corp.*, 71–1 ARB ¶8199 (1971). See also *Sahara Hotel*, 76–2 ARB ¶8410 (Koven, 1976) (drinking and drunkenness distinguished as to relative seriousness); *Packaging Corp. of America*, 56 LA 856 (Anrod, 1971) (taking drink characterized as "not extremely serious requiring immediate discharge"); *Browning-Ferris Industries of Ohio, Inc.*, 77 LA 289 (Shanker, 1981) (absent contract language making discharge for drinking mandatory, penalty for first offense depends on circumstances); and *Kaiser Sand & Gravel*, KEY CASES IN DETAIL, citing many additional authorities.

[10] *Hiram Walker & Sons, Inc.*, 3 LA 146, 148 (1946). For a more recent restatement of the same position, see *Brown & Williamson Tobacco Corp.*, 69–1 ARB ¶8478, 4625 (Stouffer, 1969): "The Union makes much of the fact that the grievant only had one drink and was capable of satisfactorily performing his job. This Arbitrator is not impressed by such argument. It could just as well be said that the Company was fortunate that it detected the grievant's drinking before he became incapable of satisfactorily performing his job or injured another employee or damaged Company equipment or property."

That the employee has no intention of getting drunk is beside the point,[11] as is (for most arbitrators) the amount[12] and proof of the beverage consumed; the plea "It was only beer!" or "It was only wine!" normally gets an employee nowhere. Arbitrator Sembower thus rejected the argument that the grievant's consumption of two beers was not really "drinking":

> "Beer in all probability is indeed 'the beverage of moderation,' but as none will deny, it is also the beverage of relaxation and conviviality. . . . [I]n light of a rule which is so clear and perfectly promulgated, there is no choice to hold that his offense is dischargeable—even in Milwaukee!"[13]

Possession of Alcoholic Beverages: The Other End of the Scale

With "possession," something at least close to unanimity of arbitral opinion finally appears. Arbitrators typically hold that merely having an intoxicant in one's possession is not so grievous a lapse as to warrant discharge for a first offense. Rules prohibiting "possession" are necessary, as one arbitrator has expressed it, since "the presence of intoxicating beverages on [company] premises could lead to the temptation to indulge in their use."[14] But where actual consumption has not taken place, the adverse consequences of mixing alcohol and work, which no-possession rules are intended to prevent, are only waiting in the wings, so to speak.

The employee who, for example, is caught with an unopened can of beer in his lunch box does not ordinarily deserve to be treated with the same severity as an employee who actually places people in danger by working while under the influence of alcohol. Some lesser discipline,

[11]As in *Brown & Williamson Tobacco Corp.*, Note 10 above: "Absence of an intent to become intoxicated while drinking on the job is immaterial; it is the violation of the drinking rule itself that is important." (at 4626) Likewise in *Diecast Corp.*, 69–1 ARB ¶8269 (Bradley, 1968), where the arbitrator sustained the grievants' discharges although they protested that it was a hot day and they only wanted to refresh themselves—not become intoxicated.

[12]*Duchess Furniture Co.*, 74–1 ARB ¶8276, 4036 (Kind, 1974): "The Arbitrator finds the amount of liquor to be of no consequence in these circumstances."

[13]*Derse Advertising Co.*, 69–2 ARB ¶8474 (Sembower, 1969). Exception has been taken to this principle in a few cases, however, e.g., in *Browning-Ferris Industries of Ohio, Inc.*, Note 9 above: "While, as earlier pointed out, the drinking of any alcoholic beverage cannot be permitted, the fact remains that more beer is needed to produce the same degree of intoxication or diminishment of control and alertness as compared to hard liquor, or as compared to the use of an illegally dangerous drug. As such, it appears that something less than the ultimate penalty of discharge might be acceptable for the drinking of a small amount of beer as opposed to the drinking of hard liquor or the ingestion of an illegal drug." (at 294)

[14]*Alcolac Chemical Corp.*, 55 LA 306 (Robertson, 1970).

such as suspension or reprimand, is considered to be more in line with that infraction.[15] And where the evidence shows convincingly that the employee had no intention of consuming the alcohol at work (despite being in possession of the beverage), no penalty at all—or at most a warning—may be in order.[16]

To Sum Up

Is it surprising, that—with the exception of "possession"—arbitrators should hold such differing views about the seriousness of alcohol violations? Not really, when two considerations are taken into account.

First: the purpose of no-alcohol rules. The underlying purpose of rules prohibiting intoxication, most everyone would agree, is to prevent certain *other things* from happening: accidents, below standard workmanship and productivity, property damage, disorderly conduct, and other harm to which intoxication may lead. (Recall Arbitrator Updegraff's comments, above). From this perspective, the real vice of intoxication lies in its potential for causing other types of problems.

To arbitrators who follow the hardest line on intoxication, the potential for harm is enough in itself to justify summary discharge. Under the same reasoning, since it too has the potential to cause intoxication, drinking calls for the same severe treatment.

To other arbitrators, "potential" is only part of the story. If no harm is done, intoxication slips down a notch. Instead of being extremely serious misconduct—the "throw him out on his ear" variety—

[15]Where the pertinent contract section provided only that employees *may* be discharged for intoxication, drinking, or possession but did not make discharge for any of those infractions *mandatory,* and where the preamble to the rules provided that the "seriousness of the offense" should be considered before discharge was invoked, the arbitrator in *Red Arrow Freight Lines, Inc.*, 78 LA 141, 144 (Baroni, 1982), decided that he had the authority to treat possession as a "lesser offense" and that "a reprimand, warning or some form of suspension should have sufficed for this first offense." Reinstatement without back pay was the award in that case, as well as in *Packaging Corp. of America,* 56 LA 856 (Anrod, 1981). The grievant received back pay in *National Car Rental System, Inc.*, 75 LA 518 (Zumas, 1980). In *Comco Metal Products, Ltd.*, 58 LA 279 (Brown, 1972), a 30–day suspension was substituted for discharge; 90 days off was the penalty in *U.S. Pipe & Foundry Co.*, 77–2 ARB ¶8479 (King, 1977). The grievants had their discharges replaced by warnings in *International Harvester, Inc.*, 23 LA 245 (Platt, 1954), and *Anvan Industries, Inc.*, 72–2 ARB ¶8516 (Kossoff, 1972) (where the contract explicitly prohibited discharge for possession without a prior warning). If the company has suspended an employee for possession, its action has generally been upheld, e.g., in *Diamond International Corp.*, 82–2 ARB ¶8326 (Ipavec, 1982) (30 days' suspension proper for bringing beer into plant), and *General Electric Co.*, 74 LA 25 (Spencer, 1979) (one week off for having glass containing whiskey in one's hand not too severe).

[16]See Chapter 2, "Reasonable Rules," p. 14, and Chapter 5, "Proof," p. 107.

it drops to very serious, but not as serious "as all that." Drinking that stops short of intoxication becomes even less serious, not only on "no harm done" grounds, but because even the potential for damage and disorder is greatly diluted when the drinker is still in control of himself.

Second: intoxication and the employer-employee relationship. To many supervisors a single episode of drinking, or even intoxication, does not inevitably brand the guilty party forever as a "bad employee." Since intoxication is neither an act of moral turpitude (like theft) nor a frontal assault on management's authority (like insubordination), many arbitrators are likewise inclined to view at least a first alcohol violation more as an unfortunate lapse of judgment than as an act of willful misconduct. This is especially so if the employee has an otherwise discipline-free record that shows him to be the kind of person who normally cares about holding up his end of the employer-employee relationship. (If his record is poor, very different conclusions inevitably must be drawn, as discussed under "Past Record and Length of Service," below.)

OTHER PENALTY FACTORS

Notice and Practice—A Dynamic Duo

Whatever the infraction—intoxication, drinking, or possession—the company can in large measure call the shots with respect to penalties *if* company rules (and in some cases the contract itself) tell employees clearly and unambiguously what penalty will be imposed for each type of infraction. This is particularly true if notice is given the "muscle" of consistent enforcement, which then becomes *past practice.* Few arbitrators will disturb a penalty, up to and including discharge, when the "rules of the game" are well known and well established.[17]

FOR EXAMPLE:

Where the company had fired every person over many years who had been found to be under the influence of alcohol, in every case using

[17]What constitutes a consistent practice may itself become a matter of dispute. In *McInerney Spring & Wire Co.*, 21 LA 80 (R. Smith, 1953), employer witnesses asserted that discharge had "always" been the penalty for bringing liquor into the plant. Only three such violations had ever come to the employer's attention, however, and the arbitrator was not persuaded that such a limited practice was enough to require the grievant's discharge in the case before him, especially since it was shown that one of the previous dischargees (unlike the grievant) had a very short work record, marked by numerous disciplinary actions, and the union had not pursued the two other cases because the grievants had lied about the facts.

the level of 0.10% blood alcohol as its definition of intoxication, the arbitrator commented: "It is difficult to conceive how a company could be more consistent in its application of a rule." Discharge was sustained.[18]

Even for possession, discharge has been sustained on a first offense where company rules warned employees in no uncertain terms that infractions would result in summary discharge,[19] or where the company has announced a concerted "crackdown" on alcohol-related misconduct of every sort.[20] The union of notice and practice has the effect of letting employees know that even if most arbitrators or most employers have other ideas, *this* company considers possession of intoxicants to be as serious as drinking and intoxication and will penalize all alcohol offenses with the same firm hand.

Conversely, if the employer has *not* put employees on notice that less serious alcohol infractions like drinking and possession will lead to discharge, many arbitrators have ruled that discharge cannot be upheld. (See Chapter 1, "Notice.")

Most employers do not follow rigid rules of disciplinary cause and effect, and for good reason. Situations have a most inconvenient way of arising where the company may find itself bound by a previously established schedule of penalties and unable to find an objective reason for deviating from that schedule. In one case where an employee reported in under the influence, the arbitrator required the company to stick to its written schedule of disciplinary penalties, which made a two-day suspension the penalty for a first infraction. Another rule that made discharge the penalty for intoxication and drinking on the premises was improperly applied.[21]

A company might also come up against a situation where a long-term, highly skilled employee commits one indiscretion and reports back after lunch one day high as a kite; assume that the company has had problems with lunchtime drinking in the past and for several years has,

[18] *Day and Zimmerman, Inc.*, KEY CASES IN DETAIL.

[19] Possessing alcoholic beverages was listed, together with drinking and intoxication, among offenses considered cause for immediate discharge in *Alcolac Chemical Corp.*, Note 14 above. In *Atlantic Steel Co.*, 50 LA 173 (Hebert, 1968), the rules stated explicitly that a first offense of possession would result in discharge.

[20] *AMF Lawn & Garden Div.*, 64 LA 988, 992 (Wyman, 1965): "Standing alone as an isolated case, discharge for the first offense of the sole act of possessing alcoholic beverages on company premises . . . might be adjudged too severe." But since the company had undertaken a well-publicized, intensive campaign to eliminate *all* alcohol-related misconduct from its premises, the grievant's discharge under those circumstances was allowed to stand.

[21] *Baumfolder Corp.*, 78 LA 1060 (Modjeska, 1980).

without exception, fired people who have shown up at work under the influence. What are its options? If it has a union, it may be able to work out an agreement that the employee can go back to work on a non-precedent-setting basis. Failing that, it either bites the bullet and lets a valued employee go; or it keeps him on and runs the risk that others will get the idea that it is getting soft on drinking, or that the next man discharged will have a winning grievance based on unequal treatment.

In summary:

The "notice and practice" combination has advantages for a company that gives a high priority to protecting itself against alcohol violations, in that the penalties it imposes have a solid chance of being upheld if challenged in arbitration. But rigidity may bind the company to certain disciplinary actions when it would rather have some leeway to take account of factors like length and quality of work record.

If, on the other hand, the company wants flexibiliity in fashioning penalties appropriate to individual situations, it gives the arbitrator greater flexibility to decide whether its judgment in particular cases conforms to the criteria by which penalties are customarily evaluated.

Presence (or Absence) of Additional Misconduct

An important consideration in weighing penalties in alcohol cases is whether the employee has aggravated his alcohol-related offense by engaging in some other misconduct. Occasionally, "drinking only" may be combined with some other infraction, as in a case where the grievants were also guilty of "flagrant absence from the job while [they] left the warehouse to purchase intoxicants. . . . "[22] But compounded misconduct crops up for the most part in cases of intoxication, which can easily lead to inability to do the job, insubordination, profanity, damage to company property, or sleeping.

***SUPPOSE:** Going too far*

Harry Workman reports to work drunk, refuses Miles Foreman's direction to go home, and uses threatening and abusive language both to foreman and to the assistant plant manager about female and black employees and about management.

[22]*Specialty Paper Box Co.*, 51 LA 120, 126 (Nathanson, 1969).

The outcome: The arbitrator finds that these additional acts of misconduct seriously aggravated the original offense of reporting for work intoxicated, so that Workman would have merited harsher treatment than other employees, who had merely been sent home when they showed up for work under the influence.[23]

One important *caveat,* however: The additional misconduct with which an employee is charged must, of course, be *proved.*[24] It must be *genuine misconduct* that could stand on its own as an offense warranting discipline. The fact that an employee is intoxicated does not automatically mean that everything he does when he is in that condition contributes to his "crime."

FOR EXAMPLE:

In *Tulsa Trailer & Body, Inc.,* 76–2 ARB ¶8450 (Williams, 1976), the arbitrator was not convinced that the insubordinate and disruptive behavior with which the grievant was charged was as serious as the employer claimed, since the foreman admitted that he did not feel threatened or intimidated and no one came up with any evidence that the grievant had interfered with anyone else's work.[25]

[23]*Libby, McNeill & Libby,* 40 LA 717 (Davis, 1963). The grievant's disruptive and abusive behavior was also found to support discharge in *White Pine Copper Co.,* 63–2 ARB ¶8548 (Larkin, 1963); while in *Monsanto Chemical Co.,* 1975 ARB ¶8235 (Casselman, 1975), the fact that the grievant, while intoxicated, threatened two foremen with a knife amply justified the 60–day suspension and year's probation that the company imposed. In *Okonite Co.,* 74 LA 664 (Ghiz, 1980), the arbitrator found that intoxication plus insubordinate conduct normally would justify discharge; only the fact that the incident took place on the last night before a vacation shutdown, when a holiday spirit prevailed and others also were celebrating, led him to commute discharge to suspension. See also *Mohawk Rubber Co.,* 47 LA 1029 (Teple, 1966) (intoxication that led to sleeping); *Combustion Engineering, Inc.,* 80 LA 503 (Heinsz, 1983) (distruction of company property); *Houston Coating Co. Div. of AMF Tuboscope, Inc.,* 68–1 ARB ¶8215 (Hon. 1968) (abusive conduct toward plant guard).

[24]For example, in *Armstrong Rubber Co.,* 77 LA 775 (Koven, 1981), the case for discharge fell apart because the company failed to prove that the grievant had threatened a supervisor or, because of his alcohol-diminished capacity, damaged the tire machine on which he was working.

[25]The arbitrator took the position that some allowance should be made for the common tendency of a drunk to deny his drunkenness: "Neither is [the arbitrator] persuaded that an employee should be penalized for arguing that he was not under the influence when it was obvious to all that he was. To find to the contrary would seemingly result in a theoretical discussion, impossible of determination, over which was 'cause' and which was 'effect.' " Management overreaction to supposed "threats" is common in intoxication cases. In *Armstrong Rubber Co.,* Note 24 above, even if the grievant stated that he would "cause trouble" for his foreman if disciplinary action were taken against him (which he denied), he could have meant only that he would pursue his remedies through the union; no physical violence was threatened. Similarly, in *Delta Refining Co.,* 79 LA 197, 82–2 ARB ¶8395 (Saracino, 1982), the arbitrator evaluated the words "you'd better get back on days, it's not safe out here at night" as "one of those unfortunate remarks often made in frustration" and not as an actual threat of violence.

Tulsa Trailer makes another important point: If the company itself "aids and abets" the grievant, by negligence or otherwise, discharge may well not stand up. In *Tulsa,* the arbitrator found that the grievant would not have had an opportunity to cause further problems were it not for the foreman's "good nature . . . in overlooking [his] arrival at work in a condition of being under the influence of alcohol" rather than sending him home immediately.[26]

By the same token, the absence of additional misconduct has sometimes worked in the grievant's favor. That "no evidence was presented that his condition affected his performance" served to mitigate the grievant's offense in one case,[27] while in another case discharge was set aside in part because the grievant, who had violated the rules by drinking in a local bar while in company uniform, was off duty and not scheduled to drive for eight hours; did not disrupt the company's schedule; and created no disturbance at the bar.[28]

Safety Factors

If an employee's job carries with it unusually hazardous working conditions, alcohol violations of any description are much more serious. The potential for alcohol-related problems is so much greater than in the ordinary case that summary discharge has often been upheld, as in the mining industry, where in one case the arbitrator commented that "what might be considered in other industries to be a rather hard nosed approach to problems of employee intoxication appears to be reasonably justified here. . . ."[29]

In the transportation industry, discharge is ordinarily regarded as a proper penalty for a driver who violates the rules against the use of

[26]Similarly, in *Libby, McNeill & Libby,* Note 23 above, the arbitrator found that the aggravating incidents would not have occurred if the company security guard had not given the grievant access to the plant, knowing full well he was drunk. That partial responsibility for the grievant's misconduct on the company's part led the arbitrator to reinstate him, although without back pay.

[27]*Standard Beverage, Inc.,* 52 LA 989 (Koven, 1969).

[28]*Greyhound Lines, Inc.,* 77–1 ARB ¶8153 (Larkin, 1977).

[29]*Consolidation Coal Co.,* 82–2 ARB ¶8605, 5703 (Sass, 1982) (discharge for on-the-job intoxication upheld). See also *Magma Copper Co.,* 64–2 ARB ¶8439 (Roberts, 1964); and *Asarco, Inc.,* 76 LA 163 (Grooms, 1981). Safety factors also made discharge proper for drinking in *Derse Advertising Co.,* Note 13 above, since employees routinely worked on high scaffolds and ladders; and in *Cities Service Co.,* 77 LA 1180, 1184 (Brisco, 1982), where the arbitrator noted that "the Company's ore processing facility with its open tanks, moving machinery, and metal grating walkways and stairs is full of hazards, especially for a person who is not fully in command of all her faculties."

alcohol.[30] Even long service may not help the grievant if sufficiently persuasive safety factors are involved.

> *Arbitrator Hebert:* "Naturally one has sympathy for one who has 15 years of service in the position of X—, but this is not basis for setting aside the discipline the Company has seen fit to impose. This plant which runs hot steel is not a setting in which to temporize with the application of rules relative to alcohol and the threat it poses to the safety of the employees."[31]

"Notice and practice" sometimes put in an appearance here. It is no accident that industries where alcohol use is especially risky are the most likely to enact rules making discharge mandatory for alcohol violations and to enforce those rules strictly, and "notice and practice" factors often join with safety factors to justify discharge penalties.[32]

Past Record and Length of Service

In cases where none of the foregoing factors is present (i.e., notice and practice, compounded misconduct, or safety factors), the variable that plays the leading role in determining the proper penalty for alcohol-related misconduct is the employee's past record and length of service.

It has become solidly established that, in one arbitrator's words, "the purpose of discipline, short of discharge, is to attempt rehabilitation of the employee so that discharge will not be necessary."[33] Under commonly accepted principles of corrective discipline, "rehabilitation"—getting the employee to mend his ways—is achieved by imposing a disciplinary suspension or at least a formal warning to get across to the employee that future misconduct will not be tolerated and will lead to more severe sanctions.

[30]E.g., in *Deluxe Saw & Tool Co.*, 70–2 ARB ¶8639 (Hon, 1970); *Humko Products*, 80–2 ARB ¶8456 (Thomson, 1980); *Farm Stores, Inc.*, 83–2 ARB ¶8447 (Hanes, 1983); *Walgreen Co.*, 66 LA 443 (Larkin, 1976); *Pacific Greyhound Lines, Inc.*, 25 LA 709 (Lennard, 1955); *Maule Industries, Inc.*, 66–2 ARB ¶8507 (Black, 1966). For an exception, see *Giant Eagle Markets, Inc.*, 1975 ARB ¶8145, 3608 (Emerson, 1975); "[I]t is a fallacy that 'progressive discipline,' as some arbitration cases have held, has no application where the operation of industrial machinery or motor vehicles is involved. Its suspension characteristic is entirely valid."

[31]*Atlantic Steel Co.*, 50 LA 173, 177 (1968).

[32]E.g., in *Atlantic Steel Co.*, Note 31 above; and *Alcolac Chemical Corp.*, 55 LA 306 (Robertson, 1970), in both of which the grievants' discharges were upheld for simple possession of alcohol.

[33]*The Taylor-Winfield Corp.*, 66–2 ARB ¶8406 (Stouffer, 1966).

Management has a special concern about the future conduct of an employee who has violated its alcohol regulations. This time, the employer might say with reason, we caught him before any damage was done; if there's a "next time," we might not be so lucky. How, then, to decide when an employee is a good bet not to hit the bottle again?

On the plus side of the ledger

Whether an employee is a good bet is determined most frequently by looking at the grievant's past record.[34] If an employee has been around for a long time, and has made a good record for himself, he is usually considered to be entitled to some "credit" for those years of service.

> *Arbitrator Gerber:* "Long service creates a presumption that the employee is capable of satisfactory performance, so that stronger evidence is needed before the contrary is established. Moreover, the senior employee has developed a greater equity in his job, which is thought of as a species of property right. He has more to lose when he is terminated and finds it more difficult to get readjusted. It is almost universally accepted that an employer must be willing to put up with more from a long service employee."[35]

Following the principle that an employee who has performed creditably in the past is a reasonable risk for the future and on that basis deserves another chance, arbitrators have reduced the discharge penalty (usually reinstating the grievant but withholding back pay as a disciplinary measure) in many cases involving intoxication,[36] as well

[34]"Thus, the principle of prediction suggests that the appropriate inquiry for the Arbitrator is to determine whether what the employee had done shows that he cannot fulfill, or will not be able to fulfill, his side of the employment bargain in the *future*." (*Arcata Graphics*, 83–1 ARB ¶8127, 3580 (Curry, 1983))

[35]*Pacific Telephone & Telegraph Co.*, 73 LA 1185, 1192 (1979).

[36]E.g., *McInerney Spring & Wire Co.*, 21 LA 80 (Smith, 1953) (four-year unblemished record); *Delta Refining Co.*, 82–2 ARB ¶8395 (Saracino, 1982) (two years with no discipline or warnings); *Kaiser Sand & Gravel*, KEY CASES IN DETAIL (four years with perfect record); *Armstrong Rubber Co.*, 77 LA 775 (Koven, 1981) (13 years with only one three-day suspension for leaving work area without permission); *McCormick & Baxter Creosoting Co.*, 55 LA 1274 (Jacobs, 1971) (11–year unblemished record, excellent attendance); *United Parcel Service*, 72 LA 1069 (White, 1979) (two-year flawless record); *Continental Can Co.*, 68–2 ARB ¶8785 (Dworkin, 1968) (10 years without discipline).

as drinking[37] and possession of alcohol.[38] A good past record of several years' duration has weighed heavily enough to justify reinstatement even in some "safety" and "compounded misconduct" cases where the grievant's fall from the straight and narrow was so evidently out of character that repetition appeared exceedingly unlikely.[39]

Sometimes, room for a "hunch"

A certain amount of intuition sometimes enters into decisions about penalty in cases where the seriousness of on-the-job intoxication and an employer's need to deter others from drinking must be weighed against the desirability of retaining a good employee and the probability that he will shape up if put back to work.

> *Arbitrator Edelman:* "Sixteen years of good service, four or five of them in a position of unusual responsibility, with no previous disciplinary action is more likely to be an accurate predictor of future performance than this one drinking incident.
>
> "It was clear from the testimony of [the grievant] as well as that of his supervisor that [the grievant] realizes full well the seriousness of his actions. He is not the kind of man who is likely to repeat the incident, but if he should, a future incident could still be dealt with."[40]

Arbitrators shy away from deciding cases on the basis of such "intangibles" as an individual's character or whether he comes to the witness stand with promises to reform flowing like wine. Pleas by the

[37] *Packaging Corp. of America,* 56 LA 856 (Anrod, 1971) (no discipline in 11 years); *Industrial Plastics Corp.,* 58 LA 546 (Willingham, 1972) (20–year record of excellent attendance, competent performance); *Greyhound Lines, Inc.,* 77–1 ARB ¶8153 (Larkin, 1977) (20 years' satisfactory service); *Great Western Chemical Co.,* 52 LA 672 (Koven, 1969) (three years with one warning letter); *Wagner Electric Co.,* 57 LA 10 (Erbs, 1971) (29½-year unblemished record).

[38] *International Harvester Co.,* 23 LA 245 (Platt, 1954) (seven years with no prior discipline); *Packaging Corp. of America,* 56 LA 856 (Anrod, 1971) (5½ years without prior discipline); *Diamond International Corp.,* 82–2 ARB ¶8326 (Ipavec, 1982) (16 years' good service justified company's decision to reduce penalty from discharge to 30–day suspension).

[39] Thus in *Libby McNeill and Libby,* 40 LA 717 (Davis, 1963), the fact that the grievant had 27 years' seniority, the last 20 of them without incident, was a major factor in the arbitrator's decision to rescind the grievant's discharge for intoxication, even though he had refused to leave the plant, caused considerable disruption, and used profanity towards other employees and management representatives both. In *Pacific Telephone & Telegraph Co.,* 73 LA 1185 (Gerber, 1979), the grievant's eight-year unblemished record persuaded the arbitrator to reinstate the grievant, even though, when a supervisor first suspected he was intoxicated and spotted a suspicious-looking paper bag in the cab of his truck, he refused to open his truck, sped recklessly out of the garage and subsequently damaged the truck. An eight-year employee was also reinstated in *Evansville State Hospital,* 69–2 ARB ¶8585 (Witney, 1969), even though the arbitrator recognized that sobriety was essential in his job as a mental hospital aide.

[40] *Southern Indiana Gas Co.,* 71–1 ARB ¶8226 (1971).

union that the penalty should be mitigated because the grievant was under great stress, had a lot of family problems, etc., rarely cut much ice either, since arbitrators acknowledge that the employer cannot as a rule be expected to bear the burden of an employee's personal problems to the extent of tolerating serious misconduct. But where the objective evidence of a long, good work record is present, indications that the grievant was going through some unusual difficulty may be an additional "make weight" factor supporting the conclusion that an outburst of misconduct was an aberration, not in his normal character and not likely to be repeated.[41]

On the negative side of the ledger

Just as a good record is customarily accepted as a predictor of good future performance, an employee's history of drinking or other misconduct may well justify a decision by the employer not to take further chances with him.

SUPPOSE: *The twice-drunk driver*

Harry Workman, a fork lift operator, was found one night in an advanced state of intoxication—he staggered, spoke with a slurred voice, and had two collisions. When confronted, he denied nothing and was sent home. Subsequently he was discharged. With Workman's misconduct a foregone conclusion, the union falls back on his history: 25 years of service and a minimal disciplinary record. Furthermore, "personal problems" Workman has been having have been "solved."

The hitch in the union's argument: About seven months before his discharge, Workman and another employee had been caught drinking and/or under the influence on the job. Workman was suspended for a week and swore it wouldn't happen again.

The arbitrator's pithy analysis: "[Workman], an obviously capable, certainly-intelligent, long-term employee, blew the deal not once but twice, and, despite that, made a really insufficient effort to either solve the problem or save his job (the same thing)." Discharge was upheld.[42]

[41]As, for example, in *Delta Refining Co.*, 82–2 ARB ¶8395, 4763 (Saracino, 1982), where the arbitrator noted, "In this case, the grievant had a good record during the two years he worked for the Company, with no previous record of discipline or warnings. All of the alleged offenses occurred on the one occasion, which may have resulted from some personal problems, of which there was some indication, but no clear definition."

[42]*Hiram Walker & Sons, Inc.*, 75 LA 899, 900 (Belshaw, 1980).

An important point to remember: Where alcohol violations are concerned, even long service may not help an employee if he comes before an arbitrator with *any* previous discipline for alcohol-related misconduct, be it a suspension,[43] or just a reprimand[44]—or, for that matter, with previous discipline for other types of misconduct.[45]

Two caveats in re past record

Caveat No. 1: For an employer to rely on the fact that an employee has been previously warned for breaking the alcohol rules, prior

[43]For example, in *Peoples Gas Light & Coke Co.*, 74–2 ARB ¶8552, 5051 (Davis, 1974), the arbitrator discounted 25 years' service saturated with warnings and suspensions for drinking on the job or showing up under the influence: "If the event of 5/14/74 had been the first instance of being under the influence of alcohol on the job, the arbitrator would doubtless have afforded the grievant another chance. The arbitrator might have done the same even if [C.] had been previously disciplined for the same offense *once* before. But the total record of the grievant, in this case, in terms of alcoholic misdeeds is so long, so overwhelming in its amplitude that there simply is no alternative in [C.'s] case to support of the Company's decision." The company need not be so tolerant; the arbitrator in *Hunt Foods and Industries, Inc.*, 64–3 ARB ¶8960 (Hebert, 1964), found that one previous two-week suspension, several months before the grievant was again caught intoxicated on the job, was enough to justify his discharge. See also *Jehl Cooperage Co.*, 75 LA 901 (Odom, 1980) (prior suspension for drinking supported grievant's discharge for possession of alcohol).

[44]Discharge was sustained, for example, in *Ocean Spray Cranberries, Inc.*, 68–1 ARB ¶8252, 3880 (Sembower, 1968), because "[o]nly about a month before the discharge, [grievant] was given a verbal warning by his foreman about his allegedly having been under the influence of alcohol on the job, coupled with a direct statement that if such did occur in the future he would be discharged." See also *Consolidation Coal Co.*, 82–2 ARB ¶8605 (Sass, 1982) (grievant previously sent home for being drunk on job and warned that another episode would lead to discharge); *Blaw-Knox Co.*, 66–2 ARB ¶8532 (Wood, 1966) (grievant previously treated leniently because of long service; warned that repetition of drinking and insubordination would mean discharge); *Ralph's Grocery Co.*, 58 LA 9 (Neblett, 1971) (grievant repeatedly warned about reporting to work with alcohol on breath, absenteeism, and other misconduct; *Chrysler Corp.*, 67–1 ARB ¶8135 (Kabaker, 1967); *Pittsburgh Steel Co.*, 63–2 ARB ¶8756 (T. McDermott, 1963).

In *Doane Products Co.*, 71–1 ARB ¶8051 (Belcher, 1970), the arbitrator specifically addressed the question whether a 10–year employee should have been suspended prior to discharge should have been attempted in the case of a 10–year employee and decided in the negative; the grievant had had ample warnings about drinking, he found, and paid no attention. Thus it was unlikely that he would respond to a suspension.

[45]*Mohawk Rubber Co.*, 47 LA 1029 (Teple, 1966) (discharge of grievant with numerous warnings and two suspensions for absenteeism, failure to report, and poor workmanship sustained, in view of many opportunities he had passed up to improve work habits); *Pacific Telephone & Telegraph Co.*, 56 LA 1191 (Hughes, 1971) (poor work record, marked by hostility towards supervision, attitude problems and customer complaints, suspension for unexcused absence, and second suspension for being outside work area, justified discharge of serviceman who drank alcoholic beverages and smoked marijuana at customer's home); *Wells Badger Industries, Inc.*, 67 LA 56, 76–2 ARB ¶8435 (J. Jones, 1976) (grievant unable to report to work because of intoxication properly discharged for excessive absenteeism); *Parkview-Gem, Inc.*, 59 LA 429 (Dugan, 1972) (discharge for intoxication upheld where grievant had record of customer complaints and other warnings about work); *American Airlines, Inc.*, 46 LA 737 (Sembower, 1966) (warnings and suspensions for absenteeism).

warnings must have been sufficiently *explicit* and *"official";* the fact that the company has "talked to" the employee informally about past incidents may not count with an arbitrator. Three cases in point:

CASE NO. 1: *No "corrective interview"*

Evidence is produced by the company that Foreman has discussed Workman's drinking habits with him, and Foreman testifies that he warned Workman that unless he corrected his problems he would be discharged.

However, there is no evidence that "he was ever so warned by anyone with authority to discharge him in a so-called corrective interview of which a written record is made, according to the usual practice. . . ." Discharge was overturned.[46]

CASE NO. 2: *"Not in those words"*

Workman was "talked to" about his drinking within a month of his discharge. "When asked, however, if he had ever told Grievant that he would be fired unless he stopped drinking, [the general foreman] replied, 'Not in those words.' " Discharge was overturned.[47]

CASE NO. 3: *The incident that got away*

Workman had previously been sent home for reporting with alcohol on his breath. However, no warning had been issued and no formal report of the incident made. On that basis, the arbitrator decided the incident of reporting under the influence for which he was fired was his first offense and put him back to work.[48]

Warnings may also be challenged on the ground that they were not specific about what kind of future misconduct would lead to further discipline—i.e., did not give proper "notice."

SUPPOSE: *"That's not what he told me!"*

Workman has been warned that if he comes to work again drunk or with whiskey on his breath, he will automatically be terminated. He is subsequently fired for bringing a small amount of beer onto company premises and drinking it with his lunch.

The outcome: The arbitrator decided the warning was "primarily directed at the consumption of hard liquor" and was not sufficiently specific to put the grievant on notice that drinking one beer could bring about his termination.[49]

[46]*Sears, Roebuck & Co.,* 35 LA 757 (Miller, 1960).
[47]*Ward Furniture Mfg. Co.,* 63–2 ARB ¶8826 (Boles, 1963).
[48]*Continental Can Co.,* 68–2 ARB ¶8785 (Dworkin, 1969).
[49]*Altamil Corp.,* 71–1 ARB ¶8199 (Volz, 1971).

Caveat No. 2: A deplorable past record will in no way justify the discharge of the grievant if the company fails to prove him guilty of the last act of misconduct which finally ended his employment.

***SUPPOSE:** Long overdue?*

Harry Workman had been sent home several times for reporting to work under the influence; was frequently absent and tardy due to drinking; had had his wages garnished—in short, according to the company, had racked up "about the worst personnel record" of all its employees. Therefore, when he showed up at work one day seemingly under the influence, the company decided it had had enough and discharged him.

The problem: True, the arbitrator agreed, Workman's record was terrible. But whether Workman really was guilty of the offense that triggered his discharge was another matter. The evidence indicated that Workman had had something to drink before reporting to work, but many of his symptoms of "drunkenness" could have been caused by a painful injury to ankle and leg.

"An employer may not . . . discharge an employee solely on the basis of prior infractions in the absence of subsequent conduct warranting some form of discipline. In short, the imposition of a penalty cannot be made retroactive unless a new cause or basis for discipline is presented."

Since that "new cause" was not proved in Workman's case, he was reinstated with one-half back pay.[50]

II. THE CHRONIC ALCOHOLIC

Where the company favors discharge as the way to deal with the chronic alcoholic, the issue that confronts the arbitrator customarily is not whether a disciplinary offense has actually been committed—since the grievant often admits his misconduct or, if he does not, his guilt is established without great difficulty. The central issue is whether the employee's alcoholism is *a mitigating circumstance* that warrants giving him another chance.

Probably the most important factor in determining the appropriate penalty is whether the particular alcoholic employee is a "first offender" who has not yet asked for or been offered help in rehabilitating himself; or whether alcohol has landed him in serious disciplinary trouble before.

[50] *Magnavox Co.*, 29 LA 305, 311 (Dworkin, 1957).

THE "FIRST OFFENSE"

If an alcoholic employee who has not taken steps to control his drinking has been discharged, arbitrators are divided as to whether alcoholism should be accepted as a mitigating circumstance. The two schools of thought are the *"too late" school,* which says "no": and the *"one more chance" school,* which says "yes."

"Too Late" School

An employee who suffers from chronic alcoholism should be afforded an opportunity to rehabilitate himself, by taking sick leave for medical treatment or by other accepted means. *But:* If the employee does not himself make an effort to get treatment *before* drinking leads to misconduct and ultimately to discharge, adherents of the "too late" school hold that an arbitrator must decide whether his discharge was for just cause according to the same criteria that he would apply to any other employee. An employee cannot, after the fact, expect an arbitrator to direct the company to give him an opportunity to rehabilitate himself.

***EXAMPLE:** Misconduct by any other name*

Harry Workman is discharged for excessive absenteeism under a contract provision which states that excessive absenteeism, regardless of the reason, can lead to termination. *The union informs* the company at the third step that Workman is a chronic alcoholic and argues that, since alcoholism is a disease, he is entitled to another chance in order to rehabilitate himself.

The arbitrator put the issue squarely:

"There is no dispute that Grievant was guilty of excessive absenteeism and that if he had been a normal healthy individual, the company would have had cause to discharge him. Does the fact that he was a confirmed alcoholic, which fact was shown to have not been made known to the company until after his discharge, be sufficient to extend to him amnesty from his excessive absenteeism."

His conclusion: Even the union agreed that Workman's attendance record was one of the worst in the industry. The company had properly warned him what would happen if he did not improve and applied the steps of progressive discipline outlined in company rules. Discharge was sustained.[51]

An employee has even less chance of getting a reprieve from a "too late" arbitrator if the evidence shows that, somewhere on the way to discharge, he was offered help by management (or the union) and rejected it.[52] Even if he has obtained help following his termination, post-discharge improvement comes too late, according to this view, and is irrelevant to the issue whether there was just cause for discharge.[53]

"One More Chance" School

Other arbitrators disagree with the foregoing approach. They take the view that because alcoholism is an illness from which it is possible to recover, discharge should not be upheld if the possibility of rehabilitation exists, even if an employee took no steps in that direction before he found himself out on the street.

EXAMPLE: *Not a virtue, but . . .*

Harry Workman is discharged for repeatedly violating a rule requiring absent employees to call the company within four hours of their starting times. *The union contends* that Workman's violations were due to his problems with alcohol, in part brought on by his estrangement from his wife, and that for those reasons, he should be given the opportunity to rehabilitate himself.

[51] *Armstrong Furnace Co.*, 63 LA 618 (Stouffer, 1974). A similar ruling was made in *Eastern Airlines, Inc.*, 74 LA 316 (Turkus, 1980). The employer had adopted specific guidelines for acceptance into an alcohol rehabilitation program. An employee who reported for work intoxicated and then asked to enroll in the program was turned down and discharged. "Too little, too late," the arbitrator ruled, finding that to grant the employee's request would amount to giving him "one free shot" in which he could show up for work drunk and escape penalty.

Other cases in this line include *Continental Airlines, Inc.*, 75 LA 896 (M. Ross, 1980); *Johns Mansville Products Corp.*, 76 LA 847 (Kates, 1981); *Western Gear Corp.*, 74 LA 641 (Sabo, 1980); *General Electric Co.*, 72 LA 355; *Du-Co Ceramics Co.*, 63 LA 655 (Wagner, 1974); *Koppers, Inc.*, 79–2 ARB ¶8613 (Lewis, 1979).

[52] As in *Johns Manville Products Corp.*, 76 LA 845 (Kates, 1981), where the grievant had previously taken a leave of absence in order to get professional help but failed to do so; *Jehl Cooperage Co.*, 75 LA 901 (Odom, 1980); *Lone Star Pennsuco, Inc.*, 80 LA 875 (Kanzer, 1983); and *NCR*, 70 LA 756 (Gundermann, 1978). In *Bordo Citrus Products Corp.*, 67 LA 1145 (Naehring, 1977), the arbitrator upheld discharge of the grievant for refusing to accept treatment for alcoholism where the grievant showed up for work intoxicated and suffered an industrial injury; had been previously suspended for drinking violations; and had been offered the opportunity to check into a hospital as an alternative to discharge.

[53] In *International Nickel Co., Inc.*, 68–2 ARB ¶8593, 5056 (Klamon, 1968), the grievant presented evidence that he had rehabilitated himself completely following his second termination for alcohol-related misconduct. Nevertheless, the arbitrator stated, "I regret that we cannot take cognizance of anything that transpired after the discharge. We can only find and hold that the discharge . . . was for just cause."

The arbitrator's view: Here too (as in *Armstrong Furnace,* Note 51 above) the arbitrator recognized that the rule Workman violated was reasonable; that he had been repeatedly warned; and that progressive discipline was followed. But the conclusion the arbitrator came to was very different:

"The violation occurred not because of an indifference toward the Company rules but because he was emotionally and physically sick. . . .

"Alcoholism is, of course, not a virtue but neither is it a wholly voluntary condition subject to the willpower of the victim. It is now fairly well recognized as an illness which affects certain people who start drinking as a social matter and find themselves gripped in its clutches. Of course, an employer is not required to put up with an alcoholic indefinitely but . . . [t]he Employer owes an employee, especially an honorable and long-standing employee, the obligation of making at least one attempt to get him to rehabilitate himself."

The outcome: Workman was reinstated (without back pay) on the condition that he continue treatment and stay out of further trouble.[54]

At the heart of this position is the view that prior warnings and progressive discipline may not have the same beneficial effect on an alcoholic as they do on other employees because of the alcoholic's notorious capacity for self-delusion about the seriousness of his problem and unrealistic belief in his ability to solve his problem on his own. It often takes something as catastrophic as what is called "the crisis of discharge" to convince an alcoholic that he needs help. Any progress towards "cure" that the employee makes following his discharge often counts in his favor with a "one more chance" arbitrator, since it is directly relevant to his "salvageability."

[54]*Armstrong Cork Co.*, 56 LA 527, 529–30 (B. Wolf, 1971). Among other cases upholding the view that an admitted alcoholic is entitled to a chance at rehabilitation, see *Monte Mart-Grand Auto Concession,* 56 LA 738, 71–1 ARB ¶8267 (1971), in which the arbitrator found that the grievant's discharge was for just cause, but gave him the opportunity to accept the employer's offer to reinstate him with seniority but without back pay if he took medical leave for professional treatment and stopped drinking. To similar effect: *American Synthetic Rubber Corp.*, 73–1 ARB ¶8070 (Kesselman, 1973); *Arcata Graphics, Buffalo Division,* 83–1 ARB ¶8127 (Curry, 1983); *Giant Eagle Markets, Inc.*, 1975 ARB ¶8145 (Emerson, 1975); *Land O'Lakes Bridgeman Creamery,* 65 LA 803 (Smythe, 1975).

In *Armstrong Rubber Co.*, 77 LA 775 (Koven, 1981); *Standard Packaging Corp.*, 71 LA 445 (Fogelberg, 1978); and *Indianapolis Rubber Co.*, 79 LA 529 (T. Gibson, 1982), the fact that the parties had an established practice of assisting employees with drinking problems added weight to the arbitrator's decision that treatment, not discharge, of alcoholic employees was called for. In *U.S. Steel Corp.*, 54 LA 760 (A. Wolff, 1970), the presence of contract language setting forth the parties' agreement to cooperate in encouraging alcoholic employees to seek treatment contributed to the arbitrator's decision to remand the case to the parties for further discussion.

Arbitrator Harter: "A number of cases show a pattern. Despite the exercise of progressive discipline by the employer, the alcoholic employee fails to respond to warnings, supervisors and other forms of discipline. When he finally exhausts the patience of his employer, he is discharged.

"During the crisis of discharge, while waiting for an arbitration hearing, he seems to pull himself together. He co-operates with those treating him, allows himself to be hospitalized, and may join Alcoholics Anonymous. By the time of the hearing his Union can point to his progress toward recovery. Authorities testify optimistically as to his prognosis."

Arbitrator Harter goes on to describe the difficult choice that an arbitrator then faces:

> "If he ignores the post-dismissal behavior and denies the grievance, he may be foreclosing all hope for the grievant. . . . Yet the arbitrator is reviewing the decision of officials as of the time of discharge. At that time they could not know what would happen between the time of discharge and the arbitration hearing."

Is there a way out of this dilemma? Harter says yes.

> "Nevertheless if the discharged employee proves after this discharge that he has a significant chance for recovery, the officials must have misjudged him and have given him too severe a penalty. The arbitrator even if he upholds the officials' charge, may reduce the penalty to give the offender a second chance."[55]

SUPPOSE: *The last one to know*

Harry Workman, a 16-year employee, has a reputation as a good worker and a discipline-free record—except for incidents involving intoxication. Prior warnings, suspensions, and counseling by his supervisors concerning drinking episodes have done no good. But the evidence shows that after discharge, he joined Alcoholics Anonymous, sought help from his church and a city alcoholic treatment center, ans was making good progress.

[55] *Pacific Northwest Bell Telephone Co.*, 66 LA 965, 972–73 (1976)

The outcome: The arbitrator accepted the union's argument that "one of the characteristic features of alcoholism is a *psychological* inability on the part of the person afflicted to face up to the rigors of rehabilitation until some drastic consequence such as discharge befalls him."[56] Workman got another chance.

By the same token, if a grievant shows convincing signs that he will not shape up, discharge may well be upheld.[57] Moreover, an employee normally will not be reinstated for the purpose of rehabilitation unless he is an alcoholic in the medical sense of the term, and not merely an individual who drinks willfully and without regard for his employment responsibilities.[58]

[56]*Chrysler Corp.*, 40 LA 935 (Alexander, 1963). See also *George A. Milton Can Co.*, 80–2 ARB ¶8561 (Handsaker, 1980); *General Abrasive Co.*, 81–2 ARB ¶8568 (Denson, 1981); *Texaco, Inc.*, 42 LA 408 (Prasow, 1963); *Standard Packaging Corp.*, 71 LA 445 (Fogelberg, 1978).

Rehabilitation, however, must be bona fide and demonstrated by tangible evidence. In *Corhart Refractories Co.*, 80–1 ARB ¶8300 (Seidman, 1979), the arbitrator found the self-serving statement of an alcoholic employee that he was "recovered" not enough, especially since he acknowledged that he still drank occasionally. In *City of Sandusky*, 73 LA 1236 (Keefe, 1979), the arbitrator refused to end the indefinite suspension of an alcoholic employee who, while still subject to a previous award requiring him to stay completely "dry," was arrested for drunk driving. In *Dahlstrom Mfg. Co., Inc.*, 78 LA 302, 306 (Gootnick, 1982), the arbitrator noted that the grievant's attendance at AA meetings had not prevented him from relapsing in the past. "Sadly, grievant has failed too often to enable this Arbitrator to conclude that his present efforts would succeed if he were again reinstated." Post-discharge rehabilitation was also not enough to persuade the arbitrator to reinstate the grievant where his job (in a mine) involved unusual hazards and it was not feasible for the employer to monitor his work closely. (*Asarco, Inc.*, 76 LA 163 (Grooms, 1981)).

[57]As in *Western Gear Corp.*, 74 LA 641, 650 (Sabo, 1980), where the arbitrator refused to believe that the grievant was sincere about rehabilitating himself when he indicated that he would seek help only in order to get his job back and "still wanted to negotiate and protect his right to drink"; and in *Continental Airlines, Inc.*, 75 LA 896 (M. Rom, 1980), where the grievant's failure to appear for the hearing led the arbitrator to doubt that he cared enough about keeping his job to be a likely candidate for rehabilitation.

[58]The arbitrator's decision in *Monsanto Chemicals Co.*, 79–2 ARB ¶8410, 4759 (Ratner, 1979), turned on the conclusion that the grievant was not an alcoholic within the medically accepted sense of the term. He observed, "It is obvious that everyone who drinks to excess or who has a hangover the next day, is not an alcoholic. . . . No employees came forward to say that [the grievant] had been noted to have alcohol on his breath. There were no traffic or driving violations; there was no evidence of family problems; there were no evidences of physical problems, as based upon the medical examination that [the grievant] received just shortly before his discharge." In short "[T]here were no objective criteria put forth to justify the contention that [the grievant] was an alcoholic at the time of his discharge. . . . "

In *Southwestern Ohio Steel, Inc.*, 1975 ARB ¶8291 (H. Dworkin, 1975), the arbitrator was not convinced the grievant suffered from genuine alcohol addiction where he appeared to drink heavily only on weekends and to be able to control his alcohol intake.

The Two Schools—a "Compare and Contrast"

By way of conclusion, arbitrators of the "too late" school differ from those of the "one more chance" school *on three fundamental questions:*

(1) *Who has the initiative for getting the alcoholic to straighten out—the employer, or the employee himself?*

According to the "too late" school, it is the individual employee who is responsible for recognizing his drinking problem and voluntarily taking the necessary steps to get help. The company's role is essentially passive; the employee himself is responsible for setting the rehabilitation process in motion, but if he does so the company usually will be obliged to give him a reasonable opportunity to straighten out.[59]

Most proponents of the "one more chance" school assign the company more responsibility for getting the alcoholic employee to seek treatment.

> *Arbitrator Kesselman:* "I generally agree with Arbitrator Walsh in an unpublished opinion that before an employee should be disciplined for alcoholism: a) he must be fully informed of the nature of his illness; b) he must be directed or encouraged to seek treatment; and c) he must refuse such treatment."[60]

The implication of this view is that management not only needs to play an active role in counseling known alcoholics but also has to be on the lookout for signs of alcoholism in employees whose drinking problems have not yet surfaced. In the larger context of the seven just-cause criteria, that means that the company may be held to special obligations with respect to both Investigation and Notice where alcoholic employees are concerned.

(2) *What counts more—the past or the future?*

The focus of the "too late" school has been described as retrospective and punitive. It focuses exclusively on what the grievant did or failed to do in the past, and disregards anything he may have done

[59]See *Warner & Swasey Co.*, 78–2 ARB ¶8370 (Siegel, 1978), where the arbitrator held that the grievant's discharge for excessive absenteeism was not for just cause since the reason for his latest period of absence (which triggered his discharge) was his voluntary self-commitment to an alcohol treatment hospital. *St. Joe Minerals Corp.* 73 LA 1193 (McDermott, 1979), and *Damascus Steel Casting Co.*, 80–1 ARB ¶8188 (J. Duff, 1980), have similar facts and outcomes.

[60]*American Synthetic Rubber Corp.*, 73–1 ARB ¶8070, 3278 (1973).

since the moment of discharge when the clock stopped insofar as his employment was concerned.[61] To the "one more chance" school, on the other hand, what is important is the future and whether there is a reasonable chance that the grievant can become a useful employee if he is put back to work.

(3) *What kind of remedy power can an arbitrator properly exercise?*

Arbitrators for many years have debated how much freedom they can properly exercise in fashioning remedies that are not specifically proposed in the parties' submission agreement or for which there is no explicit support in the contract.[62] "Two late" school decisions typically reflect the view that an arbitrator's remedy power is limited in scope and that if the contract does not provide for an alcoholic's post-discharge rehabilitation, the arbitrator would be exceeding his authority to direct such rehabilitation.[63]

"One more chance" arbitrators take the broader view that they have inherent power and that it is proper to provide remedies that may require the grievant, for example, to attend meetings of Alcoholics Anonymous; to place himself under a doctor's care; to admit himself to an alcoholic-care hospital; and/or to swear off alcoholic beverages

[61]"Some Arbitrators in dealing with these cases [involving alcoholic employees] believe that a retrospective and punitive focus is the appropriate approach to be taken by a neutral under a just cause provision. That is, they determine whether the employee's conduct has constituted a material breach of the bargain that frees the employer from its contractual obligations to this employee. Their opinions relate, often in detail, what the employee did that led his employer to terminate him. . . . The employer is seen as punishing the employee with discharge and the arbitrator is reviewing the punishment to see whether it 'fits the crime' " (*Arcata Graphics, Buffalo Division,* 83–1 ARB ¶8127, 3579 (Curry, 1983)).

[62]Remedy power is discussed at length in Marvin Hill, Jr., and Anthony V. Sinicropi, REMEDIES IN ARBITRATION (Washington, D.C.: BNA Books, 1981).

[63]Thus in *Armstrong Furnace Co.,* 63 LA 618, 620 (Stouffer, 1974), the lead case of the "too late" school, the arbitrator observed: "The Arbitrator's jurisdiction and authority is expressly limited in the Collective Bargaining Agreement. In Article 7, Section 1, Step 4(d), it is specifically stated that the Arbitrator 'shall only have jurisdiction and authority to interpret and apply the provisions of this Agreement insofar as it shall be necessary to the determination of such grievance when it asserts a violation by the Company of a specific provision of this Agreement.' . . . Nowhere in the currently effective Collective Bargaining Agreement or Company rules is there any provision granting amnesty for chronic alcoholism. . . ."

completely. Reinstatement may also be made on a "last chance" basis and conditioned upon the grievant's maintaining a clean disciplinary record for a period of time after he returns to work.[64]

The Two Schools—a Wrap

The "too late" and "one more chance" schools differ not so much in their respective attitudes towards alcoholism as in their underlying assumptions concerning the nature of arbitration and the role of the arbitrator. Decisions from the "too late school" typically see the arbitrator as a judge, evaluating the employer's actions in terms of narrow contract requirements.

"One more chance" arbitrators, on the other hand, tend to view arbitration as an extension of the collective bargaining relationship, and to pay more attention to the equities in particular cases.

THE SECOND (OR THIRD OR FOURTH) TIME AROUND

Arbitrators may disagree about the employee whose alcoholism gets him into trouble for the first time. But they have generally held that where an employee has been offered the opportunity for rehabilitation, and, instead of straightening out, has lapsed back into his former ways, discharge is all but inevitable. The reason is obvious: The first offender has a clean slate as far as the possibility of rehabilitation is concerned; the employee who has had his chance and "blown" it has proved himself to be a poor prospect for salvage.

> *Arbitrator Kesselman:* "It is unreasonable to expect any company to carry indefinitely an employee whose chronic overindulgence presents a potential danger to himself, fellow employees or plant equipment or who, because of his drinking problem, cannot perform his work duties in a responsible and efficient manner. The time does come when an employer may reasonably conclude that its efforts to encourage rehabilitation have failed and that prospects for substantial improvement are so slim that the employment relationship must be terminated."

[64]As Denenberg and Denenberg, ALCOHOL AND DRUGS: ISSUES IN THE WORKPLACE (Washington, D.C.: BNA Books, 1983), have pointed out, when remedies get too specific, they may become (improperly) more a matter of medical than arbitral judgment and/or may restrict employees' personal rights unnecessarily. To avoid such problems, they suggest that arbitrators make the terms of "conditional" reinstatement as broad as reasonably possible, e.g., by directing that the grievant be reinstated at such time as he demonstrates to the employer that he has undertaken treatment through a responsible treatment center or program and continues to participate in such program on a continuing basis (at 11–14).

In this case, the employer had twice withdrawn discharge decisions to encourage the grievant's rehabilitation, allowing medical leave and other benefits, and before the latest discharge for intoxication had put him on final notice that he was being given one last chance to cope with his drinking problem.[65]

Arbitrator Klamon: "The Company has been more than tolerant in view of the overall poor work record and the repeated incidents of intoxication of the Grievant while on duty. . . . Management in this case is not operating a hospital facility or a rehabilitation facility; nor can the Company be obliged without end to temporize with or tolerate evident chronic alcoholism. . . . "[66]

Arbitrator Larkin: "[W]hile we recognize that alcoholism is a disease, it is an illness which the patient alone can cure."[67]

SUPPOSE: *The last mile*

Harry Workman, an 11–year employee, is discharged for being drunk on the job. About five years before his discharge, he received a suspension for coming onto company premises intoxicated and engaging in an altercation with a company secretary. A few months later he was again suspended for being intoxicated on duty. He was reinstated to work on the condition that he would seek help in solving his drinking problem, and did see a doctor several times for that purpose. Testimony is introduced that he had shown up with alcohol on his breath several times thereafter—but none of his fellow employees "turned him in" until the incident which led to his discharge.

The outcome: The company had been lenient enough with Workman; his discharge was sustained.[68]

Arbitrators have come to the same conclusion in many cases where the grievant had resisted the company's efforts to turn him around or

[65]*American Synthetic Rubber Corp.*, 73–1 ARB ¶8070 (1973).

[66]*International Nickel Co., Inc.*, 68–2 ARB ¶8593 (1968).

[67]*Caterpillar Tractor Co.*, 44 LA 87 (1965).

[68]*Hughes Air Corp.*, 76–1 ARB ¶8169 (Wyckoff, 1976). Similar circumstances were present in *General Dynamics*, 79 LA 182, 184 (Rule, 1982), where the grievant was returned to work after a previous discharge for alcohol-related absenteeism. After a short period of improvement, his attendance again deteriorated as he continued to drink, and he was discharged a second time. The arbitrator was sympathetic to his declaration that he had finally admitted to himself that he was an alcoholic, but pointed out, "The mitigating circumstances which led to one reinstatement may not be used a second time when Grievant didn't do his part when he had the opportunity."

Cases of the same type include *Bethlehem Steel Corp.*, 54 LA 1090 (Porter, 1970); *U.S. Steel Corp.* 63 LA 274 (Dybeck, 1974); *Dahlstom Mfg. Co., Inc.*, 78 LA 302 (Gootnick, 1982).

was unable to control his drinking even with professional assistance.[69] There are few exceptions to the principle that an alcoholic may get one chance—but not two—to get on his feet. Such exceptions usually involve employees of very long service for whom some hope of rehabilitation still remains.[70]

It is important to bear in mind, however, that the misconduct which provokes the final discharge must be genuine misconduct. An employee's past history with alcohol may encourage a supervisor to elevate suspicion to certainty when the employee seems unusually slow one morning and has bloodshot eyes. Needless to say, jumping to conclusions is not the same as *proving* that the employee is "drunk again."

III. THE ARBITRATOR AND THE PENALTY

WHAT IF ONE OR MORE OF THE SEVEN TESTS HAVE NOT BEEN SATISFIED?

Let's assume that in imposing discipline for alcohol-related misconduct, the company satisfies all of the seven tests. Obviously that's the end of it because the just-cause scenario has been satisfied and the discipline imposed will not be disturbed, whether it be discharge or suspension or a reprimand or a warning.

If drinking, intoxication, or possession has not been proved, however, the company's entire case falls apart and the penalty it imposed, whatever it was, is invalidated. In short, no misconduct, no penalty. But

[69]The grievant's discharge was upheld in the following cases: *U.S. Military Traffic Management Command,* 75 LA 968 (Friedman, 1980) (grievant continued to be frequently absent and to report for work under the influence, despite four-year participation in an employee assistance program); *U.S. Steel Corp.,* 77 LA 854 (Hales, 1981) (grievant referred twice in two years to alcohol rehabilitation program, yet misconduct continued); *National Gypsum,* 73 LA 228 (G. Jacobs, 1979) (grievant subject to alcoholic seizures that endangered himself and fellow workers continued to have problems after dropping out of treatment program).

[70]A notable instance is *Thrifty Drug Stores, Co., Inc.,* 56 LA 789, 71–1 ARB ¶8299 (Peters, 1971), involving the discharge of an employee who "fell off the wagon" and reported to work drunk. The employee had been given two leaves of absence in one year, and was hospitalized during one of those periods. In his favor, however, was a 23–year employment history, during which he had no disciplinary problems except those having to do with his drinking; in fact, he had been repeatedly commended for his work. Moreover, the physician treating the grievant for his alcoholism testified that he was making progress, despite some backsliding. He was reinstated on a last-chance basis.

The grievant's 27 years of service also counted heavily with the arbitrator in *Pacific Northwest Bell Telephone Co.,* 66 LA 965 (Harter, 1976); while in *City of Buffalo,* 59 LA 334 (Rinaldo, 1972), the arbitrator reinstated the grievant in consideration of her 15 years' tenure and excellent work record apart from occasional drinking episodes.

let's say the company has ample proof of the grievant's culpability but falters on one or more of the six other tests. Then what? For example, what if the company failed to give proper or adequate notice of what would be the penalty for bringing intoxicants into the plant? Or it failed to conduct either an adequate or a fair investigation? Or it had neglected to enforce its no-alcohol rules consistently and without discrimination? Or suppose the company failed to observe the grievant's due process rights? Does the grievant, despite his contribution to the difficulties which befell him, go scot free?

THREE FLAVORS IN THE CREAMERY

An arbitrator has three possible choices of remedy when because of its delinquency in respect to any of the just-cause tests the company's disciplining of a culpable grievant becomes "unjust":

- *Full back pay.* The union almost always seeks in any type of discipline case that the grievant be "made whole" for all wages and other benefits he has lost as a result of his unjust discharge.
- *No back pay.* The company typically pushes this remedy if the grievant is to be reinstated at all.
- *Some back pay.* This remedy sometimes is favored by the arbitrator as a compromise between the two extremes of full back pay and none at all.

In the special case of chronic alcoholics, the arbitrator also has another option, "conditional reinstatement," requiring the grievant to get medical treatment or psychological counseling for his drinking problem, attend AA, or take other steps to get his drinking under control.

If the penalty in dispute is something less than discharge, the arbitrator has the following options:

- *Disciplinary suspension*—rescind, reduce, convert to a warning;
- *Warnings*—remove from the grievant's record, convert written warning to oral warning.

"WHAT, THEN, SHALL THE REMEDY BE?"

In the exceptional case—full back pay. Full back pay has been awarded by arbitrators in a few cases of alcohol-related misconduct, e.g., where supervisors had led the grievant to believe that drinking was condoned (failure on the Equal Treatment test)[71]; where the grievant had not been told in advance that drinking on his lunch hour was prohibited (a Notice violation)[72]; where the grievant had not been told before he agreed to take a blood alcohol test that a BAC level of 0.14 percent would be taken as conclusive proof of intoxication (Notice again)[73]; where the grievant had not had a fair chance to defend himself prior to discharge (Investigation)[74]; where the company violated the grievant's "due process" rights[75]; where the contract itself prohibited the arbitrator from imposing a lesser penalty if just cause for discharge was not found.[76]

Some back pay—a somewhat more frequent choice. Some back pay has been the choice of remedy in a number of alcohol cases where the arbitrator concluded that some penalty should be imposed, but not as severe a penalty as complete denial of back pay. What that lesser penalty should be is often dictated by the contract itself or by company rules; for example, where the grievant has been found guilty of possession of alcohol, rather than drinking, and the contract or company rules prescribe a particular penalty for possession (such as a warning or suspension of a specified length), arbitrators have normally followed that prescription.[77]

[71]As in *Luck Mining Co.*, 69–1 ARB ¶8050, 3157 (Hayes, 1968), where the grievant's supervisor had permitted employees to drink in the past: "I cannot condone Grievant's conduct, but it is my judgment that under the circumstances of this case it is justifiably excused." Company violations of both the Equal Treatment and Notice tests led to a full-back-pay award in *Industrial Plastics Corp.*, 58 LA 546, 548 (Willingham, 1972), where supervisors let the grievant drink beer on several occasions and let him know they were aware of his actions without warning him that his job was in jeopardy. "I do not condone nor approve of consumption of alcohol on the job. . . . It is also improper to knowingly permit such improper conduct for a week and suddenly discharge an offender without some attempt to correct his deficiency after 20 years plus of service to the company."

[72]*Universal City Studios, Inc.*, 65 LA 193 (Weiss, 1975).

[73]*Northrop Worldwide Services, Inc.*, 64 LA 742 (Goodstein, 1975).

[74]*U.S. Steel Corp.*, 55 LA 677 (Wolff, 1970)

[75]*Abex Corp.*, 79–2 ARB ¶8614 (Fitzgerald, 1979), where the arbitrator took a "minority" position, holding that the grievant could not be penalized for exercising his Fourth Amendment right to refuse to let a supervisor search a package that he believed contained beer. In *General Telephone of California*, 78 LA 793, 82–1 ARB ¶8198 (T. Roberts, 1982), the grievant's 10–day suspension was revoked because the company had not advised her of her right to have a union representative present when she was first questiond concerning a lunch-time drinking incident.

[76]*Conner Mfg. Co.*, 63 LA 1102 (Mulhall, 1974).

[77]As in *National Car Rental System, Inc.*, 75 LA 518 (Zumas, 1980), and *Anvan Industries, Inc.*, 72–2 ARB ¶8516 (Kossoff, 1972); back pay for time off was awarded in both cases. In *Baumfolder Corp.*, 78 LA 1060 (Modjeska, 1982), discharge was rescinded and a two-day suspension substituted where the grievant was found guilty of reporting under the influence but not of bringing alcohol onto the premises, a dischargeable offense under the company's rules.

In other cases, where the grievant's discharge has been nullified because another employee received a lesser penalty for the same offense, arbitrators have often reduced the grievant's penalty to whatever discipline the other employee received.[78] Where neither rules nor practice offers any guidance, arbitrators seek to settle upon a remedy that would seem to them to be "reasonable under all the facts of the case."[79]

The most popular flavor in the creamery. But in the great majority of alcohol cases (too many to cite here), where the proof demonstrates that the grievant was drunk, or drinking, or in possession of alcohol, but just cause was not satisfied because the company fell down on one of the other just-cause tests, the remedy has been reinstatement with no back pay. Many arbitrators opt for this remedy as being less arbitrary than a lesser penalty that may not fit in with the company's established disciplinary practices. Arbitrators often go this route on the theory that once the grievant engaged in *any* misconduct, he automatically signed on for what happened to him thereafter, including loss of work time while the case wended its way to arbitration.

The no-back-pay option has its critics, however. Some arbitrators have pointed out, for example, that if the grievant's misconduct was not really serious, the loss of earnings which results from a no-back-pay award may be a penalty that is disproportionate to the offense, especially if there has been a long delay between discharge and reinstatement.

[78]The grievants were given suspensions of the same length as their drinking companions had received in *Page Aircraft Maintenance, Inc.*, 56 LA 860 (Geissinger, 1971), and *Anaconda Co.*, 80–2 ARB ¶8380 (Cohen, 1980). In *Labor Standards Ass'n, Gimbel Brothers*, 61–3 ARB ¶8899 (Di Leone, 1961), where the instigator of a drinking party was suspended for one month, the arbitrator decided that the grievants, who had merely participated in the party, should receive lesser penalties and reduced their 30–day suspensions to one week.

[79]See, e.g., *McCormick & Baxter Creosoting Co., KEY CASES IN DETAIL* (four-week suspension, not discharge, reasonable for intoxication, in view of grievant's past record, lack of notice, and unequal treatment); *Northwest Airlines, Inc.*, 56 LA 837 (Wyckoff, 1971) (two-month suspension more appropriate than discharge for first violation of rule prohibiting drinking within 24 hours before shift); *U.S. Pipe & Foundry Co.*, 77–2 ARB ¶8479 (King, 1977) (90–day suspension proper where possession of alcohol, but not drinking, proved); *Angelica Corp.*, 62 LA 1227 (Bryan, 1974) (grievant not on notice that off-premises drunk-driving arrest would lead to discharge; 60–day suspension substituted); *Genest-Midwest, Inc.*, 67–2 ARB ¶8569 (Allman, 1967) (grievants' long service together with lax enforcement of drinking rules made one-week suspension for intoxication reasonable); *Aerojet Liquid Rocket Co.*, 75 LA 255 (Wollett, 1980) (60–day suspension substituted for discharge where company not consistent in disciplining employees who showed up for work under the influence). In *Taylor-Winfield Corp.*, 66–2 ARB ¶8406 (Stouffer, 1966), the grievant's five-day suspension for on-the-job intoxication was reduced to three days, where the grievant had a good work record and the arbitrator was convinced that three days off would be a sufficient penalty to correct his behavior.

FINAL CHECKLIST

Intoxication, Drinking, and Possession of Alcohol

The following are the principal questions that come up with respect to alcohol-related misconduct and the seven just-cause tests. If the company can answer "Yes" to these questions, the seven tests have been satisfied and discipline is for just cause. One or more "No" answers, on the other hand, may lead an arbitrator to reduce the grievant's penalty, or even rescind it.

I. Notice

In re: Misconduct

- Is the company's case free from either of the two problems that occasionally arise with respect to Notice and alcohol, i.e.:
  - Lack of notice that off-premises drinking, when it does not directly affect the employer's business, is subject to discipline?
  - Lack of notice that an employee may be required to submit to a blood alcohol test when intoxication is suspected and/or that a particular blood alcohol level will be used by the company as proof of intoxication?

In re: Penalty

- If the penalty imposed is discharge, and especially if the misconduct in question is drinking or possession, have employees been placed on advance notice that discharge can result from those offenses?
- If the rules require a specific penalty for the type of offense committed, has that penalty been imposed?

II. Reasonable Rules

- Has the rule been reasonably applied?
- If the employee's drinking or intoxication has taken place off company premises and on his own time, is his conduct covered by one or more of the "seven critical conditions" that justify discipline for off-premises misconduct?

III. Investigation

- Has the company conducted an adequate investigation according to the following three basic criteria:
  - Have all potential witnesses been questioned?
  - Has all relevant physical and documentary evidence been obtained?
  - Has the investigation been conducted in a timely manner—especially important where intoxication is suspected?

IV. Fair Investigation

- Has an investigation been conducted by some higher management official who can evaluate the evidence from the perspective of a fair and objective third party?

V. Proof

- Has the company proved that the employee committed the offense with which he is charged?
  - Intoxication—by direct and/or physical evidence?
  - Drinking—by direct and/or circumstantial evidence?
  - Possession—by direct and/or circumstantial evidence?

VI. Equal Treatment

- Has the company enforced its no-alcohol rule or rules consistently by disciplining all known violators?
- Have similar penalties been imposed for similar violations?
- If the employer seeks to penalize an employee more severely than it has penalized other people in the past, can that "unequal treatment" be justified by any of the following factors: different work records; aggravated misconduct; greater responsibility; greater job hazards; guilty intentions (in possession cases)?

VII. Penalty

- Is the proposed penalty in line with the seriousness of the offense—intoxication, drinking, or possession of alcohol?

- If the proposed discipline is discharge, is one or more of the following factors present that support that penalty: "notice and practice"; the presence of additional misconduct; safety factors; a poor past record?

(If none of these factors is present, and especially if the employee has a long and creditable past record, arbitrators have often found that discharge is too harsh and that some lesser penalty is called for—even in the case of intoxication.)

The Chronic Alcoholic

(The more "Yes" answers, the stronger the case for discharge under most circumstances.)

- Has the employee's alcoholism led to employment-related misconduct—either "short-term" (e.g., on-the-job intoxication) or "long-term" (e.g., excessive absenteeism, substandard performance)? (See Chapter 2, "Reasonable Rules.")
- Has the employee been in trouble before because of his drinking? (See Chapter 5, "Penalty.")
- Has the employee previously been given an opportunity to rehabilitate himself and then relapsed into further misconduct? (See Chapter 5, "Penalty.")
- Has the employee been allowed the same chances for rehabilitation as the company has given other alcoholic employees? (See Chapter 6, "Equal Treatment.")

APPENDIX A
KEY CASES
With Key Topics Covered

INTOXICATION

Armstrong Rubber Co., 77 LA 775 (Koven, 1981)

- Direct evidence proves intoxication
- Additional misconduct not proved
- Long service mitigates discharge
- Equal treatment of employees required

Result: Grievant reinstated without back pay

Cal Custom Hawk, 65 LA 723 (Ross, 975)

- Direct evidence of intoxication accepted
- Adverse inference from employee's refusal to take blood alcohol test

Result: Discharge upheld

Capital Area Transit Authority, 69 LA 811 (Ellman, 1977)

- Direct evidence of intoxication rejected
  —Conflicting testimony of supervisors
  —Confusion of "intoxication" symptoms with employee's normal behavior
- No prior notice that blood alcohol test would be required—no adverse inference from employee's refusal
- Lack of fair investigation

Result: Grievant reinstated without back pay

Charleston Naval Shipyard, 70–1 ARB ¶8301 (Kesselman, 1970)

- Review of arbitration cases—intoxication
- Direct evidence of intoxication accepted
- Long service mitigates penalty

Result: Grievant reinstated without back pay

Continental Can Co., 76–1 ARB ¶8006 (Sembower, 1975)

- Direct evidence of intoxication rejected
  —Supervisors overlook symptoms when grievant reports to work
- "Medication defense" accepted

Result: Grievant reinstated; back pay denied because of grievant's failure to notify company about his medication

Day & Zimmerman, Inc., 75 LA 699 (Sisk, 1980) (see also KEY CASES IN DETAIL)

- Direct evidence and blood alcohol test together prove intoxication
- Notice of penalty clear
- Discharge penalty consistently enforced
- Penalty reasonable, given "safety factors" in the grievant's job

Result: Discharge upheld

Freightliner Corp., 79–1 ARB ¶8300 (Ross, 1979) (see also KEY CASES IN DETAIL)

- Direct evidence accepted
- "Medication defense" rejected
- Lax enforcement of alcohol rules—"crackdown" notice inadequate
- Unequal penalties for alcohol violations

Result: Grievant reinstated without back pay and with "final warning"

General Felt Industries, Inc., 74 LA 972 (Carnes, 1979)

- Direct evidence—accepted symptoms reviewed
- Direct evidence rejected
  "One symptom" problem
- Interpretation of blood alcohol test results

Result: Grievants reinstated with back pay

Greif Brothers Corp., Seymour & Peck Division, Charlotte, N.C., 79–1 ARB ¶8244 (Whyte, 1979) (see also KEY CASES IN DETAIL)

- Direct evidence of intoxication
  —Absence of expected symptoms
  —Confusion of "intoxication" symptoms with grievant's normal behavior
  —"Opportunity factor"
- Refusal to take sobriety test justified—no notice of test requirement
- Poor past record does not justify discharge where no proof of present misconduct

Result: Grievant reinstated with back pay

The Holliston Mills, Inc., 73–1 ARB ¶8177 (Simon, 1973)

- Direct evidence of intoxication
  —Conflicting testimony of supervisors
  —Expected symptoms of intoxication not present
- Blood alcohol test evidence
  —Inconsistent application of standards
  —Procedural errors

- "Fumes defense" accepted

Result: Five-day suspension rescinded

Kansas-Nebraska Natural Gas Co., 40 LA 717 (Helbling, 1963) (see also KEY CASES IN DETAIL)

- Direct evidence of intoxication rejected
  —"Opportunity factor"
- "Illness defense" accepted

Result: Grievant reinstated with back pay

Libby, McNeill & Libby, 40 LA 717 (Davis, 1963)

- Misconduct compounded by employee's disruptive behavior
- Appropriateness of different penalties
- Effect of long service record

Result: Grievant reinstated without back pay

McGraw-Edison Power Systems Div., 52 LA 825 (Volz, 1969)

- Definition of "intoxication"
- Direct evidence of intoxication rejected
- "Medication defense" accepted
- Drinking on the job—"opportunity factor"

Result: Grievant reinstated without back pay

Ocean Spray Cranberries, Inc., N. Chicago Plant, 68–1 ARB ¶8252 (Sembower, 1968)

- Direct evidence proves intoxication
- Discipline for intoxication does not require a written rule
- Charge of anti-union discrimination rejected
- Prior suspension for drinking supports discharge; good record of drinking companion justifies his lesser penalty

Result: Discharge upheld

Tennessee River Pulp & Paper Co., 68 LA 421 (Simon, 1976)

- Direct evidence accepted
- Blood alcohol test required by company—Fifth Amendment issues reviewed
- Interpretation of blood alcohol test results
- "Illness defense" rejected

Result: Discharge sustained

United Parcel Service, 72 LA 1069 (White, 1979)

- Inadequate investigation casts doubt on company's motives
- Direct evidence rejected

- Medication defense accepted
- Flawless past record mitigates discharge

Result: Discharge revoked; no back pay due to culpable mixing of medication and alcohol

DRINKING

Altamil Corp., 71–1 ARB ¶8198 (Volz, 1971)

- Seriousness of drinking compared with intoxication
- Intent of no-alcohol rules
- Notice of penalty required to support discharge for "minor" drinking violation

Result: Grievant reinstated without back pay

AMF Lawn & Garden Div., 64 LA 989 (Wyman, 1975)

- Daughterty's "seven questions" applied to drinking
- Direct evidence proves drinking
  —Credibility of supervisor v. employee (the "Shulman connection")
  —Employee's explanation of the evidence not credible
- "Crackdown" on drinking justifies discharge even for first offense of drinking or possession

Result: Discharge sustained

Kaiser Sand & Gravel, 49 LA 190 (Koven, 1967) (see also KEY CASES IN DETAIL)

- Circumstantial evidence proves drinking
  —Far-fetched explanation by grievant
  —Delay in taking sobriety test
- Long and creditable service mitigates discharge

Result: Grievant reinstated without back pay

McCormick & Baxter Creosoting Co., 55 LA 1274 (Jacobs, 1971) (see also KEY CASES IN DETAIL)

- Drinking proved by circumstantial evidence
  —"Opportunity factor"
- Lax enforcement of "no drinking rule"
- Discharge penalty mitigated by grievant's long service

Result: Discharge commuted to a four-month disciplinary suspension

St. Louis Diecasting Corp., 69–1 ARB ¶8163 (Erbs, 1968)

- Direct evidence of drinking rejected
- Untimely investigation

Result: Grievant reinstated with four months' back pay

Spartek, Inc., 77–1 ARB ¶8230 (R. Gibson, 1977)

- Circumstantial evidence of drinking accepted
- Different penalties for same offense justified by different prior records

Result: Discharge sustained

POSSESSION OF ALCOHOL

International Harvester Co., 23 LA 245 (Platt, 1954)

- Possession not a serious offense
- Employee entitled to credit for long service
- Rule not consistently enforced

Result: Grievant reinstated with full back pay

Jehl Cooperage Co., 75 LA 901 (Odom, 1980)

- Direct evidence of possession accepted
- Effect of past poor record
- Safety factors justify more severe penalty

Result: Discharge upheld

Philip Morris, Inc., 68–2 ARB ¶8773 (Volz, 1968)

- Intent of "possession" rules

Result: Grievant reinstated without back pay

CHRONIC ALCOHOLISM

American Synthetic Rubber Co., 73–1 ARB ¶8070 (Kesselman, 1973)

- Chronic alcoholism—General discussion
- Poor past record of alcoholic employee—rehabilitation unsuccessful

Result: Discharge sustained

Armstrong Furnace Co., 63 LA 618 (Stouffer, 1974)

- "Too late" school—employer may discharge alcoholic employee who has not voluntarily sought rehabilitation before being fired

Result: Discharge upheld

Hughes Air Corp., 76–1 ARB ¶8169 (Wyckoff, 1976)

- On the job intoxication proved
- Prior drinking incidents and refusal of employee to control his alcoholism

Result: Discharge sustained

Pacific Northwest Bell Telephone Co., 66 LA 965 (Harter, 1976)

- "One more chance" theory explained—employee may require "crisis of discharge" to get help for alcohol problem

Result: Grievant reinstated without back pay

Texaco, Inc., 42 LA 408 (Prasow, 1963)

- Post-discharge rehabilitation efforts by grievant relevant to arbitrator's decision
- Mitigating effect of long service

Result: Grievant reinstated without back pay

APPENDIX B
KEY CASES IN DETAIL

FREIGHTLINER CORPORATION, 79–1 ARB ¶8300 (Rose, 1979)

> The Company Has the *Proof* of Intoxication, *but Can't Make It "Stick"*
>
> - Proof of intoxication
>   —Direct evidence accepted
>   —"Medication defense" rejected
> - Lax enforcement of alcohol rules—"crackdown" notice inadequate
> - Unequal penalties

Statement of the Case

On December 20, the grievant stopped to talk with a group of other leadmen on his way into work. Almost immediately the foreman was called and informed that the grievant was intoxicated. After a brief meeting with the foreman, the grievant was sent home; when he came in the next day, he was fired. Employer witnesses testified that the grievant "staggered, waved his arms, slurred his speech, rolled on his heels, and smelled of alcohol."

The company has been "waging a vigorous campaign against the ravages of intoxication," and had informed the union shortly before the grievant's discharge that it intended to post a new notice warning that any employee under the influence of alcohol would be discharged.

The union agreed that the grievant's behavior might have been a little unusual on December 20, but attributed any abnormalities to the effect of medication.

Factors in the Arbitrator's Decision

Proof of intoxication

Several supervisors, none of whom had any bias against the grievant or any stake in his termination, agreed that the grievant was under the influence. Their testimony, which deserved credit, was bolstered by the grievant's own actions. When sent home, he did not protest or ask for an explanation when told, "You don't belong here in this condition." And when discharged the next day, he did not deny that he had been drinking; the steward who was present only protested that the discharge was too harsh a penalty.

Proof of misconduct was present, the arbitrator decided. But the appropriateness of the penalty was a different matter.

"Crackdown" notice inadequate

The new notice posted by the company did not set forth a "new" anti-alcohol policy, but only repeated the working rules and contract provisions already in existence. It did not announce a change in policy.

Discriminatory penalties

Under existing policy, employees were not uniformly or consistently discharged for intoxication. There were three-day suspensions, demotions, warning letters, and shift changes—sometimes for repeat offenders. The grievant had not previously been charged with intoxication.

"And it appears that the expectation among line management personnel in the instant matter was that the grievant would receive little, if any, discipline. The paint foreman testified that the line manager informed him that the grievant was 'sent home to sober up' and would return the following morning. The personnel manager testified rather vaguely that he has terminated employees for being under the influence, and has not terminated others."

Management Condonation of Drinking

Management personnel made a practice of buying drinks for employees during lunch, considerably diluting the effectiveness of the company's anti-alcohol campaign. "There appears to be some incompatibility between an anti-drinking campaign and management encouragement of drinking at a bar during lunch. This is not to suggest that such practice increases intoxication. On the other hand, it assuredly does not enhance sobriety."

The Award

Discharge was rescinded, and the grievant was reinstated without pay and with a final warning.

GREIF BROTHERS CORP., SEYMOUR & PECK DIV., 79–1 ARB ¶8244 (Whyte, 1979)

> No Proof of Intoxication *This Time*—So *Past Record* Can't Be Considered
>
> - Direct evidence of intoxication
>   —Absence of expected symptoms
>   —Confusion of "intoxication" symptoms with grievant's normal behavior
> - "Opportunity factor"
> - Refusal to take sobriety test justified
>   —No notice of test requirement
> - Poor past record does not justify discharge absent proof of present misconduct

Statement of the Case

The evidence. On the afternoon of the grievant's discharge, his leadman came to the conclusion that he was under the influence, based upon his loud talk, use of profane language, and slow work pace. He was sent to the plant manager's office, and the manager too concluded he had been drinking since he smelled alcohol on his breath, his face was puffed, his eyes were red, and he was belligerent. He told the grievant he would have to take a breathalyzer test, and the grievant refused.

Prior warnings. The grievant had been given a warning about his slow production some three months before his discharge. Less than a month previously, on the basis of a rumor that he drank on the job, he had been cautioned that in the event of any future incident he would have to take a breath test and would be fired if it was positive.

The grievant denied that he had previously had problems for anything other than work performance, but the fact was that letters of reprimand had been issued to him a year earlier in connection with an attitude problem and improper compliance with a work order.

Factors in the Arbitrator's Decision

Proof of intoxication—subjective evidence

The grievant's symptoms. The symptoms on which the leadman based his conclusion that the grievant was drunk—offensive "shop talk," loudness, and slow work performance—were evidently nothing unusual for the grievant;

the evidence showed that he was a slow worker at the best of times, and was frequently loud as well—especially when he needed assistance in performing his work. "Shop talk" was common among all the employees.

And lack of symptoms. "In contrast there was surely opportunity to have observed an unsteady walk on the Grievant's part, if such were the case, or to have observed more than normal lack of coordination in working at his machine, if such were the case. But no such evidence was tendered."

The smell of alcohol The grievant admitted he had been drinking before work, which could account for the fact that the foreman smelled alcohol on the grievant twice during the morning of his discharge. Moreover, the foreman did not report smelling alcohol on the grievant in the afternoon, when he decided the grievant was under the influence. As for the plant manager's noticing the smell on the grievant's breath in the afternoon: "[I]t appears likely that this was expected from [the leadman's] report and not an independent evaluation."

The question of time and place

The leadman was with the grievant virtually the entire workday except for lunch, and the grievant was not seen to have anything to drink at the lunch counter where he and several other employees—and supervisors—had lunch that day.

"It stands to reason that if Grievant were drinking on the job, [the leadman] at least would have testified that the odor of alcohol was stronger on Grievant after he had been away from him for short periods. But no such evidence was given."

Refusal to take breath test

Sobriety test not like "other examinations." The company relied on a contract provision giving it the right to require certain physical and mental tests and "other examinations" to justify its demand that the grievant take a sobriety test. The arbitrator decided, however, that "other examinations" might be deemed to include psychiatric examinations or sight and hearing tests in addition to conventional physical examinations.

"A sobriety test, on the other hand, is not ordinarily considered to be either a mental or physical examination. . . . It must be concluded that [the contract] does not *per se,* obligate employees to take breathalizer tests upon company request. From this it follows that there is no basis for presuming that a refusal to take a breathalizer test constitutes an admission of consumption of alcoholic beverages."

How will test be administered? "Even if it be assumed that the company's general right to maintain production and discipline were sufficient reason for requesting a sobriety test of one kind or another, there should be a showing of the circumstances under which the test is to be taken. If it is to be done after working hours, as was a real possibility in the grievant's case, does the Company's right to make the request extend to off-duty time? . . . Who is to administer the test? Does Company employ qualified breathalizer test administrators? If Company personnel are not to administer the test, can Company require an employee to go to the police station, for example, to take it?

"These questions, among others, must be answered by the evidence before a conclusion can be reached that the breathalizer test is a reasonable means of maintaining production and discipline."

The grievant's record

Even if the company's evidence was credited and the union's evidence was disregarded, a reasonable doubt remained that the grievant was intoxicated or drinking on the day in question. Thus, the arbitrator found it unnecessary to consider either the grievant's prior warnings or possible "impeachment" of his testimony.

The Award

The grievant was reinstated with back pay.

KAISER SAND & GRAVEL, 49 LA 190 (Koven, 1967)

Grievant's *Far-Fetched Story* Does Him in—But the *Penalty* Is Another Matter

- Circumstantial evidence proves drinking
  —Far-fetched explanation by grievant
  —Delay in taking sobriety test
- Long and creditable service mitigates offense

Statement of the Case

Two empty bottles. Around 11:00 A.M. the grievant, who had been dispatched to an off-premises job site an hour earlier, was spotted in front of a liquor store by the plant superintendent. When he returned to the yard at about 12:15 P.M., the assistant superintendent checked the cab of his truck and found two small empty port wine bottles. At about the same time the grievant was talking with the dispatcher, who noticed the odor of wine on the grievant's breath. However, neither the superintendent nor the assistant superintendent reported smelling alcohol. The grievant was discharged a few minutes later for drinking on the job—though not for being under the influence.

The abortive blood test. The grievant then left the plant to arrange for a blood test, but stopped first to take care of some business at the bank and the Motor Vehicle Department, then went to the union hall and ultimately to the police station. He also stated that he visited a doctor's office at one point during the afternoon, but the doctor was not in.

The grievant's story. When the grievant was asked why the wine bottles were in his truck, he first denied their existence and then denied that they were his. Later he said he had the bottles because he intended to use one for storing diesel oil and the other for storing lemon juice at his home bar.

At the arbitration hearing he testified that he found the bottles in a ditch earlier that morning. He stated that he had had nothing to drink that morning, but he had been eating a salami and cheese sandwich (which the dispatcher testified was still unwrapped when the two were talking in the yard). He had stopped at the liquor store for tobacco, he said, not liquor. Some time after the discharge, a company representative visited the liquor store and purchased a similar kind of wine; the two bottles were packed in the same manner as the bottles found in the grievant's truck. However, neither the union nor the company went back to the store on the day of the discharge to check out the grievant's story.

No time for tippling. The union also argued that the grievant would have had little opportunity to drink two full bottles of wine (even small ones) between 11:00 A.M. and 12:15 P.M., since the contractor for whom he worked for about 45 minutes during that period submitted a written statement that he had not been drinking and the remaining time was taken up with travel to and from the job site.

The grievant's history on the job. The grievant was a 6½-year employee with a good service record, no formal complaints, and a five-year safe-driving award to his credit. The dispatcher testified that when he had been a driver, he had seen the grievant drink on the job several times but had never reported it, and the company testified that he had been told "on numerous occasions" that drinking was not permitted and that he could be discharged if proof that he was drinking was ever found. The grievant admitted on cross-examination that he had been cautioned by the plant superintendent that he was not to drink at work.

Factors in the Arbitrator's Decision

Proof of drinking—circumstantial evidence

In a nutshell, the "chain of circumstances" on which the company's case depended held up; the grievant's explanation for those circumstances did not.

Some facts are clear. "The simple fact of the grievant's situation is that he did visit the liquor store and that two empty wine bottles were found in the cab of his truck. Those facts produce a strong case against him particularly when buttressed by the dispatcher's testimony that he smelled an odor of alcohol on the grievant's breath."

The grievant's story, however, is not. "In juxtaposition to the Company's simple case against him, however, the grievant's explanation follows a tortuous path. In order to conclude that he did not drink the wine, not only must the grievant's complicated story be credited in its entirety (such as the involved conditions under which he found the bottles and the special uses for which he says they were intended) but the discrepancy between what he originally said to the Company on the intended use of those bottles ("for decorative purposes") and what he later said ("to store lemon or lime juice") must be ignored."

No time? As for the union's "no time" argument, the arbitrator found that there was no way of determining that he had no physical opportunity to have been drinking between 11:00 A.M. and 12:15 P.M., and that the union's claim that he could not have drunk both bottles of wine without becoming visibly drunk was plausible, but not *necessarily* valid.

Delay in arranging for sobriety test

The grievant's "dilatory conduct" in arranging a blood test bolstered the conclusion that he had been drinking, in the arbitrator's view. "The circuitous and involved route which he took inescapably leads to the impression that the grievant was playing for time in order to dilute the effects of the alcohol, or at the least, that he was not deadly serious about disproving the charge. . . ."

Mitigation of penalty—effect of past record

Although the preponderance of the evidence convinced the arbitrator that the grievant had been drinking on the job, nevertheless he agreed with other arbitrators that for a first offense of drinking, discharge was too severe. No formal record had ever been made of any previous drinking incidents, and the grievant was a long-service employee with a good record.

Four criteria. Moreover, reinstating the grievant without back pay would satisfy criteria for reducing the penalty in drinking cases as set forth in *Pacific Greyhound Lines,* 25 LA 709 (Lennard, 1955):

(1) No showing was made that the grievant irreparably damaged the company's confidence in him (since his misconduct was only a first offense);

(2) In view of the grievant's good work record, and in the absence of any showing that he was "incorrigible," he might reasonably be expected to correct his conduct;

(3) No aggravating circumstances were present, nor was the morale of other employees shown to have been damaged;

(4) Under all the circumstances, the penalty was harsh and unreasonable.

The Award

The grievant was reinstated, but without back pay.

KANSAS-NEBRASKA NATURAL GAS CO., 72–2 ARB ¶8493 (Helbling, 1972)

A Thorny Problem of Proof: *Anatomy of an "Illness Defense"*

- Direct evidence of intoxication rejected —"Opportunity factor"
- "Illness defense" accepted

Statement of the Case

The company's case

Drunk on arrival. The grievant worked the midnight to 8:00 A.M. shift and was the only employee on duty during those hours. At about 12:15 A.M. on August 18, the plant superintendent received a call from the employee whom the grievant had just relieved. He told the superintendent that the grievant appeared to be intoxicated when he reported to work.

Passed out on the job. Together with the plant engineer, whom he had called, the superintendent found the grievant at about 1:00 A.M. in the calorimeter building, a building with neither windows nor telephone located about 200 feet from the grievant's normal work location. The grievant was lying with a rug folded beneath him and his shoes unlaced, sleeping. The superintendent and engineer detected the odor of alcohol. They left and returned with a mechanic about half an hour later and awakened the grievant, who said he felt unwell.

Symptoms of intoxication. The superintendent testified that the grievant appeared to be intoxicated, "that he walked in a very deliberate manner with occasional meandering steps; that he had difficulty walking over several pipes, and that the engineer also believed the grievant was drunk." He was told to go home.

Subsequent events. On August 19 the personnel manager conducted an investigation of the foregoing events, questioning the superintendent, engineer, mechanic, and the employee who had initially reported the grievant's intoxicated state. He tried to reach the grievant on that date but could not. The grievant was subsequently suspended.

On August 20 the grievant met with the superintendent at the plant and explained that he had been ill the night of the 18th; that he lay down with the hope of feeling better and planned to call the superintendent if he did not. On the grievant's authorization, the superintendent learned that day from the grievant's doctor that the grievant had telephoned the doctor's office at about 9:30 A.M. on August 18th and requested some medication of a type he had had for a prior illness, but had been told that he would have to be examined first. The superintendent again spoke with the doctor on August 23, after the grievant had been examined, and was informed that the grievant was suffering from high blood pressure which might cause him to pass out.

The grievant was discharged on August 24 on the ground that he had been intoxicated the night of August 18.

The union's response

Nothing to drink. The grievant testified that he had spent the 12 hours before reporting to work on the night in question repairing an acquaintance's TV set—except for about 20 minutes traveling time from his acquaintance's home to the plant. That he had nothing to drink during that 12–hour period was confirmed by the TV set's owner.

Seizure—then blackout. At about 12:15 A.M. he had begun to experience the same symptoms he had had three years earlier—he felt shaky and weak and then blacked out and experienced rapid changes of heat and cold. He stated that he telephoned the superintendent's number, heard a male voice that he assumed was the superintendent's, and told him he was sick. He could not recall anything further until he was awakened. With respect to his shoes, he said he often left the laces loose.

The smell of alcohol. After being sent home he had driven himself home and called the union. A union representative had come to his house at about 2:00 A.M.; the representative later testified that the grievant did not appear intoxicated. He also testified that the company kept industrial alcohol on the premises, which smells much like alcoholic beverages.

Factors in the Arbitrator's Decision

Proof of intoxication—the "illness defense"

The issue was clear: Were the grievant's symptoms the night of August 18 produced by intoxication or illness? The medical evidence established that the grievant did indeed suffer from a physical condition that *might* have caused the symptoms he exhibited that night. But *did* it? The problem was that "the direct evidence so closely supports opposing contentions on that issue."

The "scene of the crime." "On its face, the evidence that the grievant was found in a building which had no telephone and which was a substantial distance from the office where he made a phone call, raises the inference that the grievant chose a place where he would not likely be found. Moreover, the presence of a folded rug beneath his head fits into the argument that the grievent sought to 'sleep off' his intoxication." But "since a resolution of this dispute must rest on which probability, i.e., sickness or drunkenness, was the causal factor, consideration must be given to *what might have reasonably occurred if the grievant was ill"* (emphasis added). If the grievant was indeed suffering from a seizure, he "may have been subject to the kind of physical and emotional disorientation which impeded the exercise of sound judgment," so that his choice of a fairly remote location to lie down does not *necessarily* weigh against him.

The "meandering steps" and other symptoms reported by the superintendent are consistent with symptoms of intoxication; but they are also "consonant with a condition in which a person is revived after feeling vertigo." Though the smell of alcohol detected by the superintendent and the engineer had some probative value that the grievant was intoxicated, neither one testified that he smelled alcohol on the grievant's breath. That industrial alcohol was present in the plant was not disputed, and it was not shown that no alcohol was present in the calorimeter building on the evening in question.

To the doctor right away? The company argued that the grievant's failure to go immediately to the doctor or the hospital suggested that he was not as sick as he claimed. The arbitrator found that reasoning "plausible but short of being persuasive" in view of the grievant's testimony that he felt better after he left the plant and telephoned the doctor first thing in the morning to request medication.

What else could the company have done? Two pieces of evidence which *might* have established that the grievant was under the influence, and not sick, on the night of August 18 were not produced by the company.

First, the individual who was in the best position to have determined whether the grievant was intoxicated was the employee who first observed his condition—the employee who telephoned the superintendent. But that employee was not called to testify, and his hearsay report was given little weight. The company pointed out that the union attorney had interviewed this employee. It claimed that if the grievant were innocent, the union would have called him to testify. But the arbitrator held that the argument cut the other way: It was the company that had the burden of proof, and its failure to call the employee was even more harmful to the company's case.

Second, although the best time to have proved whether the grievant was intoxicated was "on the spot," no attempt was made to have the grievant take a sobriety test. Under normal conditions a sobriety test might not be necessary, but here the grievant stated that he did not feel well. Moreover, the superintendent himself knew that the grievant had suffered a seizure at the plant three years earlier—indeed, he had helped get him to the hospital. Under these circumstances, the superintendent might reasonably have been expected to try to obtain "objective" confirmation that the grievant was intoxicated.

The question of time and place

Workman's testimony that he had had nothing to drink during the 12 hours before he reported to work was corroborated by the owner of the TV set he had been working on. It is true that he could have drunk something in the 20 minutes it took him to get from his acquaintance's house to the plant; but such an inference must be evaluated according to the physical manifestations of intoxication—which were none too clear.

The arbitrator's final conclusion: stalemate

"A full evaluation of the record produces the conclusion that the evidence which supports the charge of drunkenness is counterbalanced by testimony which weighs in favor of the contention that the grievant was ill. But, in order to sustain the discharge, the Company had the burden of presenting a case which preponderates in its favor." That the company did not do.

The Award

The grievant was reinstated with back pay.

MCCORMICK & BAXTER CREOSOTING CO., 55 LA 1274 (Jacobs, 1971)

Empty Bottles and an Angry Wife—*Drinking Proved, but Discharge Ruled Out*

- Drinking proved by circumstantial evidence —"Opportunity factor"
- Lax enforcement of "no-drinking" rule
- Discharge penalty mitigated by grievant's long service

Statement of the Case

The grievant had been employed for 11 years at the time of his discharge. During that period he received no warning notices about drinking or any other misconduct, and his only discipline was a two-day disciplinary layoff five years earlier for leaving for lunch two or three minutes early. His attendance was excellent. The company's work involved handling large loads of lumber and working with heavy equipment, and was classified as very hazardous.

An "overpowering" odor. The grievant was discharged for drinking on the job after the Yard Superintendent went to where the grievant was working at about 2:00 P.M. to move him to another job. While the two men were riding in the Superintendent's pick-up truck, the Superintendent noticed the "overpowering" smell of liquor and subsequently told Foreman what he had observed and asked him to keep an eye on the grievant to see if he noticed the same thing.

Empty bottles. Later in the day, Foreman reported to the Superintendent that he had found three empty liquor bottles in the tool shack where the grievant had been working, as well as a "cold pack" of a kind used for keeping drinks cold. Discharge followed.

Two beers at lunch. The grievant denied that he had been drinking on the job and further denied any knowledge of the bottles in the shack. He admitted having drunk alcohol on the job on prior occasions, but on the day in question, stated that he had only had two bottles of beer with his lunch. According to another employee, he had no problems handling a forklift, with whose operation he was unfamiliar, that afternoon.

A crackdown? About ten months before the grievant's discharge, three employees (including a foreman) had been caught drinking on the job and received suspensions. Shortly thereafter, a notice was posted to the effect that there would be no drinking on the job and that anyone caught would be discharged. The grievant admitted that he had read the notice.

Factors in the Aribtrator's Decision

Proof of drinking—circumstantial evidence

The "chain of circumstantial evidence" satisfied the Arbitrator that the grievant had been drinking.

In the grievant's bin. It was undisputed that the Foreman found the empty bottles and cold pack in the shed where the grievant had been working. Though it was true that other employees were seen going in and out of the shack that afternoon, the arbitrator could not accept the grievant's statement that he had no knowledge of the bottles—especially since one bottle was found in a bin containing numbers which the grievant was using in his job. He also found the grievant's statement that the "cold pack" had been there for several months, unused, difficult to credit.

Two "time and place" factors

(1) The physical evidence of the bottles was corroborated by the yard superintendent's testimony about the strong smell of alcohol on the grievant's breath at 2:00 P.M. The arbitrator did not doubt that the grievant had been drinking beer at lunch, but questioned whether those two beers, consumed two hours earlier, wold have accounted for the "overpowering" smell.

(2) Finally, the grievant's wife had previously complained to the yard superintendent that her husband was coming home from work drunk—too soon after quitting time to be accounted for by a stop-off at a bar!

Lax enforcement of anti-drinking rules

In general. Despite the posting of the "no drinking" notice, it was clear to the arbitrator that no effort had been made to enforce it. Although the yard superintendent testified that the company had had problems with other employees besides the grievant drinking at work, no employees were discharged, or even warned or reprimanded between the posting of the notice and the time the grievant was discharged.

The grievant himself. The Superintendent even reported prior problems with the grievant himself, stating that he had become "suspicious" that he was drinking on earlier occasions, because on some afternoons, his face would become red, his speech very loud, and he would smell of alcohol. Despite these observations—and despite the call from the grievant's wife—the Superintendent never explained why he did not discipline or at least warn the grievant on any prior occasion.

"While the Arbitrator is in no way indicating the actions (or lack of action) by the Company constituted a waiver or abandonment of the posted notice or rule, it must be taken into consideration in arriving at a determination whether discharge was too severe a penalty."

Effect of past record

In view of the grievant's long and generally excellent work record, as well as the lack of prior warnings or discipline for drinking—and even though dangers were involved in the company's work—the arbitrator found that discharge was too harsh a punishment.

The Award

Discharge was not sustained, but was commuted to a four-week disciplinary layoff.

DAY & ZIMMERMAN, INC., 75 LA 699 (Sisk, 1980)

Model Company Case: *Every Necessary Element Present* in a Discharge for Intoxication

- Direct evidence and blood alcohol test together prove intoxication
- Notice of penalty clear
- Discharge penalty consistently enforced
- Penalty reasonable, given "safety factors" in the grievant's job

Statement of the Case

As the grievant was reporting to work at the ammunition plant where he worked, the maintenance superintendent noticed that he "weaved and staggered somewhat" and, when he stopped to talk to him, smelled whiskey on his breath. About 45 minutes later, in the presence of a union steward, the grievant voluntarily took a "breathalyzer" test, which showed that he had a blood alcohol level of 0.17%. (The security officer who administered the test agreed with the superintendent that the grievant's "walking appeared to be unsteady.")

The grievant denied throughout that he had been drinking, claiming instead that he had used a mouthful of whiskey as a mouthwash.

Factors in the Arbitrator's Decision

Proof of intoxication

"The investigation prior to G—'s discharge was complete in every respect. There was the observation of his immediate superintendent. That observation is verified by the objective findings of the breathalyzer test." All that evidence—the reports of witnesses and the test results—was taken into consideration at the meeting where the discharge decision was made.

Clear notice of penalty

"There is no doubt," the arbitrator noted, "that the Company has publicized its rules for employees." The Employee Information Manual stated specifically that "[b]eing under the influence of alcoholic drinks while on the Reservation . . . *will be punished by separation from the payroll for the first offense"* (emphasis in original). And the contract itself provided that "[D]rinking of or being under the influence of alcoholic beverages or drugs while on duty or drinking of alcoholic beverages of Company property . . . shall be causes for immediate dismissal."

"[T]he Company has consistently used the level of 0.10% of blood alcohol as an indication that a person is under the influence of alcohol. (It is noted in passing that percentage levels of blood alcohol less than 0.10% are used as verification of the charge of having alcohol on one's breath, a lesser offense.)"

Penalty consistently enforced

The director of industrial relations testified that every employee who had been found under the influence on company premises had been discharged, and a list going back some 28 years was submitted. "It is difficult to conceive how a company could be more consistent in its application of a rule."

Penalty reasonable, given hazardous conditions.

"In view of the fact that the facility . . . is engaged in making live ammunition it must be concluded that the rule is reasonable if for no other reason than the nature of the product."

The Award

The grievance was denied "in its entirety."

APPENDIX C

ALCOHOL AND THE WORKPLACE— A BASIC BIBLIOGRAPHY

ALCOHOL AND HEALTH: NEW KNOWLEDGE (Washington, D.C.: U.S. Dept. of Health, Education and Welfare, ADAMHA, NIAA)

Andrewson, Dale E., "Arbitral Views of Alcoholism Cases," *Personnel Journal,* 58 (1979), pp. 318–22.

Choate, P. W., "Alcoholism: To Treat or Terminate—Arbitral Response," *Canadian Personnel and Industrial Relations Journal,* 27 (1980), pp. 29–34.

Daykin, Walter L., "Alcoholic in Industry," *Labor Law Journal,* 11 (1960), pp. 883–90.

Denenberg, Tia S., "The Arbitration of Alcohol Drug Abuse Cases," *Arbitration Journal,* 35 (1980), pp. 16–21.

Denenberg, Tia S. and R. V., ALCOHOL AND DRUGS: ISSUES IN THE WORKPLACE (Washington, D.C.: BNA Books, 1983).
Recent general study.

Drahn, Theodore L., "Alcohol and Working Americans," *Industrial Gerontology,* new series 1 (1974), pp. 1–19.
Includes extensive bibliography on earlier books and articles on the subject of work-related alcoholism and on-the-job drinking.

Dugan, Robert D., "Affirmative Action for Alcoholics and Addicts?," *Employee Relations Law Journal,* 5 (1979), pp. 235–44.

Godwin, Donald F., "The Problems of Alcoholism in Industry," ARBITRATION—1975, Proceedings of the 28th Annual Meeting, National Academy of Arbitrators (Washington, D.C.: BNA Books, 1976), pp. 97–103.

Habbe, Stephen, COMPANY CONTROLS FOR DRINKING PROBLEMS (New York: National Industrial Conference Board, 1969).

Hill, Barbara J., "Alcoholism and the World of Work," ARBITRATION—1975, Proceedings of the 28th Annual Meeting, National Academy of Arbitrators (Washington, D.C.: BNA Books, 1976), pp. 93–97.

Hodge, J., "The Alcoholic Employee—A Review," *Management Quarterly,* 21 (1980), pp. 14–18.

Jones, Ronald E., "Alcoholism and the Workplace," *Manpower,* 7 (1975), pp. 3–8.

Kurtz, N. R., "Managing the Alcoholic Employee," *Industrial Management,* 21 (1979), pp. 15–21.

MacDonald, James H. and P. Don Sparks, "Employee Assistance Program for Alcoholism and Drug Abuse: An Industry Approach," *Industrial Gerontology,* new series 1 (1974), pp. 25–27.

Marmo, Michael, "Arbitrators View Alcoholic Employees: Discipline or Rehabilitation," *Arbitration Journal,* 37 (1982), pp. 17–27.

OCCUPATIONAL ALCOHOLISM: SOME PROBLEMS AND SOME SOLUTIONS (Washington, D.C.: U.S. Dept. of Health Education and Welfare), Pub. No. (HSM) 73–9060.

Provost, Glendel J., et al., "Alcohol in the Workplace: A Review of Recent Arbitration Cases," *Employee Relations Law Journal,* 4 (1978–79), pp. 400–14.

Provost, Glendel J., et al., "Alcohol or Drug Use on the Job: A Study of Arbitration Cases," *Employee Relations Law Journal,* 5 (1979), pp. 245–57.

Simons, Jesse, "Alcoholism, Drug Abuse and Excessive Absences," PROCEEDINGS OF NEW YORK UNIVERSITY THIRTY-SECOND ANNUAL CONFERENCE ON LABOR, 1979 (New York: Matthew Bender, 1980), pp. 125–37.

Somers, Gerald G., "Alcohol and the Just Cause for Discharge," ARBITRATION—1975, Proceedings of the 28th Annual Meeting, National Academy of Arbitrators (Washington, D.C.: BNA Books, 1976), pp. 103–17.

Spencer, Janet M., "The Developing Notion of Employer Responsibility for the Alcoholic, Drug-Addicted or Mentally Ill Employee: An Examination Under Federal and State Employment Statutes and Arbitration Decisions," *Saint John's Law Review,* 53 (1979), pp. 659–720.

Trice, Harrison M., "Alcoholism and the Work World," *Sloan Management Review,* 12 (1970), pp. 67–75.

Trice, Harrison M., THE PROBLEM DRINKER ON THE JOB (Ithaca, N.Y.: New York State School of Industrial Relations, Cornell University, 1959).

Trice, Harrison M., and James Belasco, EMOTIONAL HEALTH AND EMPLOYER RESPONSIBILITY (Ithaca, N.Y.: New York State School of Industrial and Labor Relations, Cornell University, 1966).

Trice, Harrison M., and Janice M. Beyer, IMPLEMENTING CHANGE: ALCOHOLISM POLICIES IN WORK ORGANIZATIONS (New York: Free Press, 1978).

Trice, Harrison M., and Paul M. Roman, SPIRITS AND DEMONS AT WORK (Ithaca, N.Y.: New York State School of Industrial and Labor Relations, Cornell Univ., 1972)

A thoroughgoing survey of alcohol and drug problems at the workplace, with full bibliography of earlier sources.

Tucker, Jerry R., "A Worker-Oriented Alcoholism and Troubled Employee Program: A Union Approach," *Industrial Gerontology,* new series 1 (1974), pp. 20–24.

Worker, J. J., "Supervising the Alcoholic Employee," *Supervisory Management,* 23 (1978), pp. 26–32.

TOPICAL INDEX